the Medicine Cabinet

Byron G. Wels

HAMMOND INCORPORATED
MAPLEWOOD, NEW JERSEY 07040

Dedication

In my entire writing career I've heard about editors who actually worked closely with their authors, but never really met one. The editors I worked with would accept my manuscripts, thank me, then pay me and I never heard any further word until bound books were delivered.

Frank Brady, Editorial Director at Hammond's Trade Division, was different. He kept right on top of me and this work, was concerned over how the research was coming, helped to unearth information and sources, found authoritative consultants and made numerous suggestions to improve the text. He coaxed me, cajoled, and even insulated me from some of my more severe critics. He also knew how to administer a swift kick where and when it was needed.

It is therefore with thanks and appreciation that I dedicate this work to Frank Brady, wishing that there were more editors like him.

Byron G. Wels

ENTIRE CONTENTS © COPYRIGHT 1978 BY HAMMOND INCORPORATED

All rights reserved. No part of this book may be reproduced or utilized in any form or by any means, electronic or mechanical, including photocopying, recording or by any information storage and retrieval system, without permission in writing from the Publisher.

PRINTED IN THE UNITED STATES OF AMERICA

Library of Congress Cataloging in Publication Data
Wels, Byron G.
　The medicine cabinet.
　　Includes index.
　　1. Drugs, Nonprescription.　2. Self-medication.　I. Title.
RM671.A1W44　　615'.1　　78-5517
ISBN 0-8437-3407-8
ISBN 0-8437-3408-6 pbk.

Contents

One: Introduction	5-12
Two: Making the Decision	13-19
Three: Restocking	20-27
Four: How To Buy ... And Take ... Medications	28-39
Five: Contraindications and Interactions	40-53
Six: The Accessories	54-59
Seven: Analgesics	60-71
Recommended Adult Dosage Schedules for Standard and Nonstandard Asprin, Acetaminophen or Sodium Salicylate Dosage Units	69
Internal Analgesics	70-71
Eight: Vitamins	72-77
Vitamin Product Content Chart	74-77
Nine: First Aid	78-83
Ten: Wounds	84-88
Eleven: Burns and Scalds	89-95
Burn and Sunburn Remedies	95
Twelve: Skin Problems	96-106
Acne Preparations	98-99
Thirteen: The Mouth and Teeth	107-112
Mouthwash Ingredients	112
Fourteen: "Eye, Ear, Nose and Throat"	113-129
Fifteen: Mucous Membranes	130-135
Hemorrhoid Products	135
Sixteen: Your Lungs and Breathing	136-141
Cold and Allergy Products	140-141
Seventeen: Your Digestive System	142-169
Antacids	166-167
Laxatives	168-169
Eighteen: Muscle Problems	170-174
Nineteen: The Portable Medicine Cabinet	175-179
Twenty: That Other Family Member	180-185
Twenty-One: Charts	186-188
Interactions	187-188
Index	189-192

NOTE

The first aid, medical and health procedures contained in this book are based on thorough research and the recommendations of responsible medical sources, including that of William M. Weinstein, a community pharmacist and a Professor of Pharmacy at Rutgers College of Pharmacy.

The author, publisher and editors, however, disclaim responsibility for any adverse effects or consequences resulting from the suggestions or use of any of the preparations contained herein. The procedures and preparations described in this book are not appropriate in all cases for all individuals. Even if appropriate, they may cause harm if used incorrectly or indiscriminately.

In all cases, it is recommended that the reader check with his physician before using or consuming any drug.

Chapter One

Introduction

When a health-related crisis occurs in your family, even a small one, one of the first places you'll probably turn to will be your medicine cabinet. Unfortunately, too many people wait until a crisis develops before they equip their medicine cabinets to meet that unexpected emergency. As a result, it often is an after-the-fact catchall for whatever happens to fall into it. Should a member of the family, for example, develop a headache, you'll buy a headache remedy, then put the remainder of the medicine into the medicine cabinet until the next time somebody has a similar disorder. This hit-or-miss method of buying medications offers no assurance that sufficient medication of the type you may need will be there when you need it.

Another thing that ends up in the medicine cabinet is the prescription medication that your physician will, from time to time, prescribe for you or another family member. A child had a sore throat, and the doctor sent you the drugstore for the prescription. The child's throat improved before the remedy ran out, so what's left goes into the medicine cabinet. Who knows? Perhaps the child or another family member might develop a sore throat in the future, and — it is erroneously believed — you'll not only save the cost of a new prescription, you'll save the cost of the doctor's visit too.

Unfortunately, an inventory of the average family's medicine cabinet will reveal that the most common items are a motley assortment of cosmetics, old lipsticks, spare razor blades, aftershave lotion, deodorants and other items that are used every day and are most conveniently stored in the bathroom. A few pointed questions must be asked, although there may not be any immediate answers for them.

Many pharmacists do *not* mark prescription bottles to identify the contents. Look through your medicine cabinet at some of those bottles. Can you identify each and every bottle? Can you say — with certainty — what each was originally for? Do you know positively when it was compounded? Or the name of the medicine?

Can you be positive that the bottles of patent remedies that you have purchased and stored over the years are still sufficiently potent to do the job for which they were originally purchased?

Are you certain that the old remedies you purchased and stored, even if no longer potent, might not actually have deteriorated to a point where they may actually be harmful and may cause trouble rather than the cure you hoped for?

And finally, can you say with any degree of certainty that you are prepared and equipped to cope with any situation requiring relatively fast treatment in your own home?

"Of course I have a suitable burn ointment," you might say. But take a good look at your medicine cabinet. Do you *really* have on hand an ointment that will effectively cope with burns? Is it in a place where you can immediately find it when the need arises? Or did you just *think* you had some? If you do find it, is it fresh enough still to be good? Do you know how to apply it?

The answers to the foregoing questions and other ones is what this book is all about. The average individual is *really* in trouble when he is faced with a medical emergency. Although most people have a scant smattering of knowledge of the basics of first aid, picked up by hearsay or when they were Boy Scouts, this is hardly sufficient to cope with a serious emergency. People rely heavily on the advice of their pharmacists for the recommendation of nonprescription remedies, but there's much more than we must know, if we intend to "Be Prepared."

Consider, too, the familiar "stuffers" that accompany any and all drug items that you can buy. When you have an illness of any sort, all you want to do is get the remedy inside you so it can start working... and you can feel better again. You tear the package open, pull the medication out and take the recommended dosage. What happens to the stuffer (or as it is properly called, "the package insert")? That's probably the bit of printed paper that you threw away, complaining about the manufacturer's "advertising" that filled the box. It is imperative that you read the instructions and other information on the package insert. It may save your life.

Sometimes lessons are learned the hard way. A friend, suffering a severe head cold, asked another friend what he should take. His friend recommended one of the popular cold remedies containing a decongestant. Following the advice on the carton, two tablets were taken. The cold symptoms appeared to lessen and the stuffer was read just in time to stop taking the next scheduled dose of the remedy. People with high blood pressure should not take this remedy — it was "contraindicated," which means that it is highly inadvisable for those with high blood pressure to take.

What this book is *not* going to be, is "Your Family Medical Advisor." It is going to provide you with good, commonsense facts regarding the family medicine cabinet and its contents. It will discuss many nonprescription items that you can buy at any drug counter, tell you what the active ingredients are, what they're good for and what they aren't good for.

Hopefully, you will read the book through, then keep it as a handy reference. We intend to deal with the various available nonprescription items in relation to the maladies they are designed to correct. Antacids, for example, will be located in the chapter titled Your Digestive System.

One of the most important benefits in this book will be the charts found with many of the chapters listing many of the nonprescription drugs found on the market according to their function. We will be describing their ingredients in detail, so that if you are allergic to any of the contents, you can avoid them. You will also learn about the potency of a number of drugs on the basis of time. You will read what the contraindications or interactions are, and you will realize which of the drugs produced by one manufacturer are essentially the same as those of another manufacturer, but with a different name.

Obviously, a book such as this cannot be limited to drugs alone, for there are many other health-related devices that can be of equal importance, and these will be covered here as well. You'll find much information on stethoscopes, splints, hot water bottles and ice bags.

You'll also learn about thermometers. Did you know, for example, that the British use thermometers neither orally nor rectally, but prefer to take the temperature in the armpit? There's also a difference in the normal body temperature, depending on where the thermometer is used.

Most importantly, you're going to learn about *your* medicine cabinet. The chances are that your medicine cabinet is like most medicine cabinets; you have gathered an assortment of materials that really have little or no value in terms of emergency treatment. In our own opinion, the space alloted to a typical medicine cabinet is completely inadequate, and therefore we're going to begin by suggesting that the actual medicine cabinet itself be given completely over to the various cosmetics and sundries that have gathered therein. We're also going to suggest that a small closet — perhaps a portion of a linen closet — be devoted to the proper storage of medications in the home.

If such a closet is not available, you'll find that you can purchase a suitable cabinet that *will* find a proper place in your home. What we're looking for is plenty of shelf space for storage of small bottles, jars and vials, larger-size bottles, and plenty of vertical room for other large-size materials that may be required.

Extremely critical, too, is the need for adequate lighting in this closet. We recommend vertical flourescent lamps with suitable light shields so the light can be concentrated toward the shelves and away from the eyes to avoid glare. Flourescent lamps are recommended because they will not cast shadows as incandescent lamps will. We don't want you to have to guess when you reach for a bottle on the shelf!

You're going to want additional shelf space in this closet, so do add the necessary shelves at this time, and by all means paint the entire inside in a light, bright color. The closet door can be used for taping up such emergency information as the phone number of the local emergency or first aid squad, the local pharmacy and, of course, your physician.

Now we're going to do some evaluating of what might be on hand and still usable. Let's begin with the old bottles of prescription medications that your family did not use up. All of these should be tossed out. Prescription drugs, once prescribed for a specific illness, should not be taken again unless the physician prescribes them again. All of these should be flushed down the toilet. To save what's left, regardless of the cost, is a mistake. The drugs may have gone bad, and you'll be better off to replace them when the doctor re-prescribes them.

There is one exception. What we said applies to *acute* illnesses, those problems that come up occasionally for which medication is taken as a specific remedy. *Chronic* illnesses are another matter entirely. If your doctor advises you to take a medication over a period of a long time, and the medication is to be taken when symptoms recur (as in the case of hay fever), naturally it would be foolish to throw away the remainder of the drug and buy a new supply when the problem recurs.

Nonprescription medications can also suffer the effects of aging, and, whether liquid or solid, certain of the critical ingredients can change and lose potency over a period of time. Since the chances are that you have not indicated a purchase date on the label, it's a good idea to dispose of any of these that have not been used and replace them, if needed, with new remedies.

Few lay people are aware, for example, that the patent remedies indicate by their very name how they are compounded. A "tincture" for example, (i.e., tincture of iodine) tells you that the medication is compounded with an alcohol base. The percentage of alcohol is also included on the label. However, alcohol is a highly volatile product that will rapidly evaporate when the bottle is opened. Obviously, as the bottle is opened some of the alcohol evaporates, and the percentage changes. In sufficient time, a new supply must be obtained.

It's amazing, too, how, in their haste to apply a medication, many people will improperly replace the cap so that it is put on too loosely, cross-threaded so it doesn't close correctly, or even neglect to cap the bottle at all.

The point is that those patent remedies that you find in your medicine cabinet at this point should be carefully examined, and if any doubt exists as to age or potency, they should be disposed of at once.

Many drug items require refrigeration, and any that do that have *not* been refrigerated, should be destroyed. Before commencing on the redesign of your medicine cabinet, read the entire book and then reread and follow the recommendations on a step-by-step basis.

The importance of this is borne out (as an example) in photography, for if you buy a fresh roll of film and put it in the refrigerator, it will not age or deteriorate. It will remain fresh for as long as it is kept cold, despite the date on the film carton. Many of the drugs you'll buy are the same. Keep them cold and they'll stay fresh and potent. Let heat get at them and they will rapidly deteriorate. It's fairly obvious that gelatin capsules will melt when exposed to body temperature. If you place a bottle of medicine in capsule form in a suitcase and then put the suitcase in the trunk of your car on a warm summer's day, you're going to find a melted mess of medicine and capsules. Body temperature, at which capsules melt, is not a great deal compared to the oven-like temperature of a hot trunk.

While the gelatin capsule is merely a container for the medical dosage, some chemicals themselves can rapidly deteriorate in heat. If the label is marked for refrigeration, by all means, keep the product refrigerated.

In the next chapter, there is an evaluation of what you might already have in your medicine cabinet. You will also find an explanation of how to arrive at a safe, sane and intelligent decision about what to do with these items.

Important? Sure it is! When you reach for something to help you or a member of your family toward more comfort and safety, it should be there, ready for instant use.

Throughout this book, you're going to hear several names for the remedies that are mentioned. Let's explain them now, for they also describe the purview of this work.

"Self-medications" is the popular term in use today, for it describes those medicines that you can prescribe for yourself without a physician's written prescription form. "OTC" or "over-the-counter" drugs is another term that is often used. These medications are indeed sold "over the counter." They are fully prepared and require no compounding to prepare. The most interesting of the terms is actually an archaic one, "Patent Remedies." This goes back to Old England, where a man would discover such a remedy and receive "letters patent" from the Government to manufacture and sell the product.

Consider the old adage, "The man who is his own doctor has a fool for a patient." If you are going to prescribe your own medicines, please take the time and trouble to read the "stuffers" — those package inserts that can tell you that if you are already taking a medicine, you ought not to take the one that you may be holding in your hand!

The day of the "pill roller" is just about gone. Pharmacists today still occasionally compound their own medications, following a doctor's prescription. But for the most part, medications that are prescribed are standard, and the pharmacist merely counts them out. In the case of nonprescription specifics, even this is not done. Chances are that you will ask for such products by name and brand, and you must consider that the item has been manufactured, placed in cartons and then shipped to drug wholesalers, then to the individual drugstore. These can sit on various shelves for some time before you purchase them. As you will learn in this book, many of these are not affected by aging, and the vials or bottles are sealed with a plastic shrink-wrap that keeps them sealed. However, as a safety measure, you should always mark the purchase date on the label.

Overdosing — even on nonprescription drugs — can be a problem. This is especially true where children are concerned. Some medicines are often colorful, nicely flavored and are therefore extremely attractive to youngsters. More than once a child has eaten an entire "chocolate bar," not realizing that it was Ex-Lax chocolated laxative. Candy-coated laxatives such as Feen-A-Mint are also appealing, and because children inexplicably enjoy the taste of aspirin, serious poisoning problems can occur with these as well.

It's not always the youngster who is the victim. Any adult may dutifully take a sleeping pill before retiring, and then, when he wakes during the night, groggy with sleep, he may reach for the bottle of sleeping pills, thinking perhaps that he had forgotten to take it. This can be repeated so often in so short a time that one might overdose without realizing it.

We're going to recommend that some positive action be taken to prevent this. One way is to set up a small, lockable cabinet within your family medicine cabinet. This lockable cabinet should require a key to open it, and that key should be placed in an easily accessible location some distance from the medicine cabinet. You must actually *think* about taking a medication and simply must not just reach for it during the night.

Another suggestion is to wrap each critical container of medication in a strip of coarse sandpaper. When you reach for this bottle, you will instantly know that there is something different about it, and will, hopefully, think before taking it. If this method is used, children should be taught that the bottles with sandpaper strips on them are not to be touched.

The Medicine Cabinet is not a guide that is going to recommend a specific medication for a specific problem. There is only one person who can properly perform the functions of a physician — diagnose an illness and prescribe for it — and that is the physician himself. If you're ever in doubt, by all means consult him. What might (for example) appear to be a simple backache could be a kidney problem. Covering or masking the pain with an analgesic, a back rub or an aspirin will *not* correct the problem.

Your family medicine cabinet is something like fire, an excellent servant but a horrible master. It can be a panacea when an emergency arises, provided that you have it properly prepared and equipped to handle such emergencies. At the same time, if it or the items inside it are misused, it can be deadly dangerous.

Chapter Two

Making the Decision

Medicines can be expensive, and when a medication is needed and has served its purpose, it takes a bit of courage to throw away what might be left in the bottle. But when a physician prescribes a medication, he also prescribes the amount and expects you to consume all of it before the course of treatment is completed. If you have any left over, you have not followed your doctor's instructions. Perhaps you missed taking a dose or two, or maybe you stopped taking the medicine because you felt better. In any case leftover prescription medicines should be thrown away. While this is especially true for prescription medications, this applies to the over-the-counter medicines as well.

There are exceptions.

If you have a chronic condition that requires constant medication such as tranquilizers, hay fever medicines or blood pressure medicines that you must take regularly, you shouldn't throw the medicine away when your condition improves. But the acute problems that require specific treatment are another story. If you have a severe cough, for example, and the doctor prescribes a prescription cough medicine, you may have some left over. If one of your children then develops a cough, you might feel that this same medicine might help the child, too. You couldn't possibly be making a bigger mistake! For there are many good reasons not to do this. The cough may *not* be the same. It could be a symptom of a more serious problem that only a physician can diagnose. There may be contraindications, the dosage may be wrong, the potency of the drug too strong.

In acting as your own physician, you are doubtless doing more harm than good. Another important factor is the matter of confusion. Are you absolutely *certain* that the medicine in the cabinet is what you think it is? It may have been some time since it was prescribed, and who knows — at this point — what, or who, it was really for?

Finally, there's the expiration date, which we will be getting into in more detail later on. For a prescription medication can change in time; it can lose or gain in potency, and while in some instances it may not actually cause any harm, in others it can be harmful. And when its potency has deteriorated, there's no way that the medicine can help.

Suppose, for example, there's a medicine that has an adverse effect on the stomach. The manufacturer introduces a buffering agent to offset this. In time, let's assume that the active agents continue to have their beneficial effect, but that the buffering agents have expired. You take the medication, and you may feel both better and worse!

Which brings us to another major, important point. As stated above, a prescription medication recommended for a certain family member by a physician must either be completely consumed during the course of treatment, or, if any remains, it should be immediately disposed of. The only time that such medication can be retained for future use is on the specific advice of that physician.

What this means is that if your physician prescribes a tranquilizer such as Valium, or a pain killer such as Darvon to be taken as needed, we don't mean for you to toss away the remaining drugs after you've used them for the first time. These drugs are prescribed for chronic, not acute symptoms.

There are certain gray areas where your own good sense must rule. If you have any doubt, throw it out. If you can't decide, ask your physician.

If you think there was confusion and a lack of information where the prescription drugs are concerned, consider the problems you'll come across where patent remedies or other nonprescription items are concerned.

The average family faces a difficult decision when it comes to the purchase of patent remedies. If you buy the smallest quantity available when and as it is needed, you are assured freshness and potency each time you take the medication. If you buy these small quantities, however, you pay a great deal more, for the very packaging is expensive. Should you buy the larger quantities and effect a cost saving? Or are you better off with the smallest amounts to be sure of freshness? There's the matter of convenience, too. The larger quantities take more space, are less portable, and because they last longer, are usually subject to deterioration over a given time period.

In the "old days," people bought large quantities of such items and stored them against the time they'd be needed. For convenience, they carried small pillboxes with them, boxes of gold or platinum inlaid with ivory, and a day's supply of whatever was needed was simply slipped into a change purse or a vest pocket. Today, you can get almost any sort of medication in a small enough packet to be eminently portable. Aspirin, cold tablets or capsules — all come in small plastic packages or convenient tins. Antacids come in handy rolls. Decongestants are available in squeeze bottles or atomizing inhalers. All fit nicely into a modern purse or dispatch case.

Still, when you compare the price of the small, handy, easy-to-carry package with the huge economy bottle, you may find that the price per unit is escalated several times, just for the convenience.

How to determine what quantities to buy of which items? You are best qualified to judge your families' needs, and a study of the pattern of consumption will help you determine the quantities to buy.

If you're a single adult living alone, the chances are that the smallest quantities will serve best. Need adhesive bandages? Probably the smallest quantity of assorted types will last you well over a year. On the other hand, if you have a fairly large family of young children, you may find that cuts, scratches and bruises occur with sufficient frequency that the largest package of such bandages will scarcely last a week. Your greatest economy will come from buying the larger numbers.

Bioavailability

An important factor in determining how much of a drug product to take is what physicians call "bioavailability." This is an efficiency factor which indicates how much of a drug product will be found in the bloodstream at a given time after the drug is taken.

Bioavailability is determined by the solubility of a drug, one's own rate of absorption of the chemical, and other factors. As an example, if an aspirin tablet is taken, and then it is found that (after suitable blood analysis) there is 0.001 gram per cubic centimeter in the bloodstream after one hour from taking the tablet, then this is the bioavailibility of aspirin.

Since the rates at which drugs are found in the bloodstream vary from individual to individual, knowing your own bioavailability rate for a given drug can be more useful in determining the proper dosage than can reading the instructions on the label. Unfortunately unless you are equipped to do your own blood tests, there's no way for you to know. The best we can hope for is an averaging, and you'll learn through your own experience which ones are more effective for you.

A living-alone adult may find that he injests aspirin as if it were peanuts. The small, convenient bottle might last no longer than a week, if that long. The initial purchase of the minium quantity in the small bottle can be considered. This bottle can then be carried about conveniently and restocked as needed from a larger bottle which has been purchased for economy's sake.

Your best decision as to how much to buy can be derived by your own experience with the products in question. If your family uses a great deal of the product, buy it in larger quantities. If you use it rarely or infrequently, buy the smaller quantities.

The important thing to remember here is that you should have a minimum quantity of fresh product to be on hand when the need for it arises. Here's a typical example:

There is a product available that serves as a topical anaesthetic for the specific relief of toothache. Under ordinary circumstances, the only time you'd buy this product is when somebody had a need for it, and you couldn't get to a dentist. But it may be late at night, the dentist might not be available, the pharmacist might be closed. If you have a pain killer available, you might offer the victim a dose of that. As we all know, it isn't really going to do the trick, and you're going to wish you had the correct remedy in the house.

If, on the other hand, you had the foresight to purchase this product "just in case," you'd apply some of it to the affected areas, the victim of this siege of pain would be able to get some sleep, and so would you. The next day, a visit to the dentist would properly and permanently relieve the pain.

Preparing the Medicine Cabinet

Begin by clearing a kitchen or dining room table. Then bring all of the contents of the medicine cabinet to this place. Dispose of all the drugs that are prescription items that are no longer used on a regular basis and under a doctor's direction. Where any doubt exists, dispose of the product at once, and with no looking back or regret.

Next start on the nonprescription drugs. Dated products should not be used beyond the expiration date. If an expiration date appears on the label and that date has passed, dispose of the product. If the product is undated and more than a year old, dispose of it. Those products that are less than one year old and are to be saved must be marked with the date on which you did this work. Mark these dates right on the label so there will not be any doubt when they are needed.

How can you know how good a product is and whether or not it should be disposed of?

Creams and ointments can deteriorate quite visibly. They become hard and brittle, and the decomposition is quite noticeable. Avoid the temptation to simply "squeeze the bad part out of the tube" and use what's left. By the same token, if the surface film on such a product in a jar seems bad, do not attempt to remove the bad part and hope that the rest is still good. Chances are that certain parts of the product have separated from the rest.

Liquids can also go bad. If the product was originally an emulsion and the emulsion has broken, simply shaking the bottle and using it again will not do. Or if it has discolored or developed a strange odor, dispose of it.

Capsules should be carefully checked for integrity. If some — even one, or a few — of the capsules have broken or partially melted, dispose of the entire lot.

Tablets can also go "sour," and you should look for softness by crumbling one between your fingers. The intrusion of moisture will be evidenced by a "furry" growth on the tablets. These must also be thrown away.

Disposing of Drugs

What is the right way to dispose of drug items? Correct disposal can actually protect your family. If you drop the unwanted drugs in a garbage can, they can still be retrieved. Youngsters in your own home can still get them out of the garbage — animals can recover them. The smartest and best way is to open the packages, pour the medication into the toilet and flush until it's all gone. The empty bottles can then be deposited in the garbage.

Controlled-Dosage Medications

If you have any medications such as prescribed sleeping pills that must be taken only in limited quantities, another problem is introduced.

Controlled-dosage medications must be taken under strictly supervised circumstances, leaving nothing about timing to doubt. If you have somebody in the home that can control the timing of such medications, leave the timing to that person. When you are under such medication, you might not be thinking straight, and a well person, wide awake and alert, should be present to supervise such timing. If you take too many such medications at too frequent intervals, you may wind up facing death, or, at the very least, the added discomfort of a stomach pump.

Here are some suggestions that you may find worthwhile:

a) Place a few bands of pressure-sensitive tape around the bottle, with the adhesive side out. When you touch one of these bottles, you'll feel the stickiness, and this will cause you to realize that the bottle contains something "special."

b) A thin band of sandpaper wrapped around the bottle or its cap can have the same effect.

c) Make sure the bottle has one of those "child-proof" caps that will make you actually work at getting it off.

d) Place such medications under lock and key, in a separate container such as a small cash box or securities box, with the key in a separate place. To get at the medication, you must first locate the key, open the box, and then — and only then — can you get to the medicine. There's no chance that you'll still be half asleep, or that you can take the medicine by accident.

The question that you *must* ask when making the decision to dispose of certain products is this: "If I give this medicine to a family member, not being sure of its age or potency, can I be sure that it will provide the hoped-for relief? Will it possibly, due to its age, cause more harm than good? Can it, again because of its age, actually do damage?"

In the light of questions such as these, one must do a careful bit of soul searching before actually deciding to keep a specific remedy and save the cost of replacement.

Obviously, any rational person reading these words is going to view the situation with a certain amount of suspicion. After all, the many manufacturers and packagers of these remedies and products will be the ones to benefit ultimately if you throw away the products and replace them with fresh stock. This is true. The various packagers are interested in sales of their products, and if they could get you to throw them away and replace them instead of waiting until they are used, they would stand to benefit. But this writer has no axe to grind. He is not in the employ of these packagers, and has not been pressured by anyone to make any specific recommendations. The advice and suggestions here are his own, and nobody else's. While it may be true that ultimately the packager will benefit, do keep in mind that your own family will derive an even greater benefit.

Therefore, it is most strongly recommended that you be absolutely ruthless in making your decision. Make note of purchase dates, how much was purchased, how much has been used, and how much remains. It is on this basis that we will, in the next chapter, decide on what products will be bought for restocking, and how much should be purchased.

The most important thing to remember in evaluating the products in your medicine cabinet is that when in doubt, throw it out!

Chapter Three

Restocking

After you have organized and cleaned up your medicine cabinet you're ready to prepare yourself for any minor health crisis by restocking it. What do you buy? What don't you buy?

It's really a very personal decision. Your medicine cabinet needs will reflect the particular needs of your own family, and while you will want to stock it with those medications that your family uses in large quantities, you will also want to have those items on hand that there may be a need for in an emergency. You will want to tailor your purchases to your own family's needs, of course. But at the same time, you'll want to have additional items that visitors might need.

For example, if you have sensitive stomachs in your family, you'll want an analgesic which also has a buffering agent that can soothe and ease a tender tummy. However, you might want one of those "maximum strength, faster-acting" pain relievers that will be asked for by a guest with a severe headache seeking faster relief.

Maybe you're the sort of stoic that can withstand the sting of Merthiolate when you get a cut, but others might want an antiseptic that's a bit more gentle. Your philosophy when restocking the medicine cabinet should be to obtain a sufficient quantity of the various products that may be needed, not just for yourself, but for your family and friends as well.

Our suggestion on how to go about this business of restocking a medicine cabinet is to go through the balance of this book, making notes about those products you think you will need, and then taking the list to your pharmacist and giving him the order, asking his advice and recommendations as well. Before you do this, however, there are certain questions that must be asked and answered.

It is certainly not our intention to advise you on brand names. Nor do we plan to offer our own opinions on the value of one particular drug over another.

The Federal Government exercises tight controls on the content of patent remedies, and when a manufacturer or packager informs you, via the stuffer or label, that you're getting "so many milligrams of _____." you can be certain that this is quite correct. Should a drug product manufacturer attempt — for whatever reason — to falsify content claims that he makes, he'd be in more trouble than it could be worth.

There are several firms that package drugs under lesser-known brand names and who sell their products for a good deal less than the popular brands are sold. These "discount" drug manufacturers make use of this fact as a point in their advertising. It is their claim that because Federal regulations control the content, quantity and quality, that you might just as well buy their own brands of product, pay a good deal less, and get essentially the same benefits without having to pay for costly advertising programs that the big name manufacturers require.

Of course, there's an element of truth in this claim. And there's a fallacy here as well. The so-called "discount drug" manufacturers do, indeed, sell their products for less at times. But they also have high advertising budgets in order to bring this information to the public. They will promote what are called "loss leaders," which are certain of their items that are sold at or (in some cases) below cost to attract you to their products. You compare the price of such a "loss leader" with the price of a name-brand drug and feel that you are getting a real bargain, as indeed you are. You may be led to expect that the same low prices will apply to all products of that brand, but on examination you might find that on other items, their prices are the same or higher than the name brands. Some of the discount firms have actually grown tremendously, and they manage to compete quite nicely with the well-known "name" firms. On the other hand, the discount firm and the name-brand house both have strict quality-control systems, seeing to it that their products are carefully sampled before making their way to your medicine cabinet. But as one of them pointed out, a sampling of product does not assure you of the uniformity of the product and that the capsule, pill or tablet that you take is as good as the ones that have been tested. The tests are destructive, in that checking on a sample basis destroys the medicinal unit being tested. Of course, any testing is usually better than no testing at all, and in buying the name brands, you do have a staid, respectable firm behind the products that you buy.

What should you do with what you buy? Believe it or not, sometimes it is more involved than simply putting it on the shelf in a neat, orderly style.

If the container is airtight, or if refrigeration is required after opening, you can leave it on the shelf until the first time it is opened. By all means, check the instructions carefully. Many products contain materials that are designed to protect the product from becoming damaged during shipment. You may find a small ball of absorbent cotton when you open the bottle. This must be removed and disposed of at once! It is just there to protect the product from physical abuse. If left in place, or returned to the bottle, it can collect moisture and transfer this to the product in the container.

Other products use a silica-gel compound in a breathable paper packet. This, on the other hand, should be kept in the container until the product is completely used up. It will extract moisture from the container, keeping the moisture away from the product.

As you can determine from our suggestions, the chances are that you're going to find more than one product for each possible ailment. Because there is little or no uniformity among the manufacturers, you're going to have an assortment of bottles, vials, jars, tubes, boxes and tins. Be certain that each is positioned in such a way that the product labels clearly show from the front. Unfortunately, many of the adhesives used to attach the labels are not always reliable and under conditions of heat and humidity, these adhesives can in time release, and a crucial label will be lost. To avoid this, try applying a length of transparent self-adhesive tape around the bottle or jar to keep the label from dropping off, even if its own adhesive lets go. If you use "invisible" tape, you'll find it easy to write additional information on the label with a ball-point pen. For example, you can add the date of purchase to the container in this way.

Some medications must be protected against heat, and if so, the label instructions and/or the package insert will so indicate. Such medications must be treated like any others, but with the stipulation that they be kept under constant refrigeration.

Another thing to consider carefully when restocking your medicine cabinet is the presence of youngsters in your home. Children have little or no sense when it comes to medicines and, let's face it, those colorful liquids and capsules can, to the eye of a child, be deceiving. Anything that looks that good, they will reason, has simply got to taste good too. The kids are not always wrong, either. Since no medication can do any good until it is taken, the manufacturers indulge us by adding suitable flavorings to disguise the possibility of unpleasant taste and make the product more palatable. Since most kids don't read, they depend on association and recognition. A candy-coated laxative that so closely resembles a candy-coated chewing gum just might be evaluated by a child as chewing gum. Many well-meaning parents, having to give a child a pill to swallow, tell the youngsters, "It's a piece of candy." There's more than one case on record of aspirin poisoning or overdosing on Ex-Lax or Feen-A-Mint.

You may decide that the best route is simply to educate the child against the use of these medications. But a child's mind can either fail to grasp or twist and turn meanings, so that warnings are simply insufficient to the task. Drugs and drug-related products must be kept from children by suitable means. See the section on Controlled Dosage Medications in Chapter Two for suggestions.

Many people are reluctant to rush out and fully replenish the medicine cabinet all at once. It may be an expensive operation, to be sure, but you can do it step-by-step, starting with those products that are essentials. You can add to the larder on a regular and ongoing basis. You'll find that by purchasing a single typical product for a specific ailment, you very quickly achieve a basic supply in each area, and your medicine cabinet can quickly and easily be equipped with the proper basics, at a modest cost. Once this has been achieved, you need only add to the supply to provide diversification and completeness.

In the area of stomach specifics, for example, you'll want an antacid, a laxative, a palliative for such things as diarrhea and stomach upset, as well as one or two others for other problems that may occur frequently in your family.

The type of remedy that you select will be determined primarily by the sort that you and your family prefer — you will purchase those medications that you have learned through experience will provide the best and quickest relief. Later, as time and budget permit, you can add to these with others that might better suit visitors or guests.

Let's examine some antacids in tablet form which are available in rolls or boxes. These come with varying degrees of "chewability" and come in assorted flavors to make them palatable. Without the flavoring, they usually have an unpleasant, chalky taste. Should you prefer this tablet form of antacid, you'll be faced with a wide assortment of these alone from which to make your selection! You have to settle on a brand, then select the flavor you prefer, and as you will later learn, the content — the active ingredients — can change from brand to brand and you'll have to decide on which works best for you. It can be a morass of decision making.

If a tablet is to be used, you may find that your physician will recommend a specific one for you. By all means, do follow his suggestion.

When it comes to the effervescent forms, you'll be faced with a choice of tablets or granules. And there's more than one of each of those to choose from too! This brings to mind a situation that occurred some time ago.

One patient found that the symptoms of acid indigestion and heart attack are quite similar. The severe, constricting chest pain, the pain felt through the left arm, led him directly to the doctor's office for an electrocardiogram. The doctor prescribed a mild, yellow, triangular tablet which later proved to be a placebo — ordinary sugar tablets.

Then an "attack" occurred while visiting a relative who was a physician. He took a large, white tablet from his bag; it was dutifully chewed and swallowed, and this resulted in a long, loud belch and almost instant relief of the pain. The "heart condition" turned out to be nothing more or less than simple heartburn.

How should you go about restocking your medicine cabinet? Our own suggestion would be that you go over the charts in this book and check with other responsible family members, making a "yes" or "no" decision on each and every product, carefully listing all of the "yesses." Make a complete inventory sheet, eliminating those you decide against.

You will find certain remedies that are required for chronic problems, others designed only for acute needs. Your first choices should be the remedies that you feel you must have. The vitamins that you take regularly should also be included here, as well as the necessary analgesics, stomach remedies, etcetera.

The next items you will select will be those that are used a bit less frequently. However, these are still things that you and your family have come to depend on. Often, you and members of the family will simply feel more secure and comfortable knowing that these products are on hand should they be needed. They may include certain first aid items or toothache medications, laxatives or additional stomach remedies. They are not really necessary on a day-to-day basis, but are nice to have on hand, just in case.

Now add the products that you think you might one day require.

These are the once-in-awhile things that would be nice to have on hand, just to say to yourself that your stock is complete. In this section, you will purchase those questionable things that fall between the gray area of "maybe" and an outright "no."

Finally, make a list of those things that visitors or guests might require that are not duplicated on your own list. These are simply considerate purchases that you make for friends. When a visitor is stricken with a problem and does not have access to his own remedies, he says, "Do you have any Excedrin?" Maybe your own preference is Bufferin, but how nice to be able when a visitor asks, "Have you an analgesic," to ask in return, "What kind would you like?" When purchasing these items, always buy the minimal quantities.

The next step is to form shopping lists. Start with those in the first, most important category, then fill in with the others as time and inclination dictate. Once you have the basics on hand, the chances are that you will be able to cope with any problem that may come up. Stocking up on the next category will make you feel even more secure.

Be certain to date your purchases, put them away properly, and be sure that you carefully read all labels and insert directions.

Reading is an essential to making drug purchases. The Proprietary Association in Washington, D.C., is an organized group of pharmaceutical manufacturers. We spoke to one of the directors, who explained that his organization was concerned about the publication of this book. We explained that one of the big things we planned to do was to urge people to read and follow directions. This, it seems, is one of the Association's goals as well. We were offered all sorts of cooperation.

If you take the time and trouble to read the valuable information on the content, use and dosage of certain of these remedies you'll save yourself a great deal of grief.

In restocking your medicine cabinet, you're going to find a number of nonprescription drugs that are relatively new to you. While most new products in this field are given an excellent promotion by packagers, thereby making them at least *seem* to be familiar, others are not quite as fortunate,,and you'll be seeing them for the first time when you shop for your restock items. As different people can react differently to the same products, there's not much point in asking others who may have tried these just how efficacious they are. By all means, examine the packages and make an attempt to evaluate the active ingredients by comparing these (and the amount they contain) with others that you may know. Some of the newer medicines are complex in that they contain not only the basic active ingredient, but in addition to this specific for the problem you are trying to correct, they may contain secondary ingredients whose purpose is to counteract any adverse problems that may possibly arise as a result of the action of the active ingredient on your system.

In recent years, pain relievers without aspirin have become popular under the trade names Tylenol or Datril. These are acetaminophen compounds, a drug at least as old as aspirin. It it a different type of pain reliever which has the added advantage of not being an inflammatory. For people who cannot take aspirin, these products provide an excellent solution.

Before closing this chapter on restocking, we'd like to make one more point. Once your medicine cabinet is restocked, a routine stock taking schedule should be established in order to dispose of outdated items and to replenish exhausted or low supplies.

Chapter Four

How To Buy... And Take... Medications

If you're like most people, you find a great deal of confusion in this area. You're deluged with various brand names, you wonder whether or not you are buying the best value, and whether or not trying to save money might cost you the benefits that you hope to get from taking the medication.

You've probably heard that a patient should ask his physician to prescribe medications by the generic name rather than by a brand name — that this results in a fantastic cost saving (or it could be) to you. But what about the nonprescription drugs that you prescribe for yourself? It seems that these days the well-known, standard brands are in competition with unfamiliar off-brand or private label medications. These off-brands are usually sold on the basis of price, and often have names that seem to mimic the better-known brands that are probably familiar to you.

It's an interesting — and factual — point that all medications are strictly controlled as to content of active ingredients by the Pure Food and Drug laws. By law, these packagers are not permitted to alter arbitrarily formulations or content, must maintain purity, and must comply with the same, stringent regulations with which the better-known packagers are forced to comply. Well, if the contents of the bottle are the same, if the only difference is in the name, why aren't the better-known packagers forced by reason of economics to reduce their prices? The larger packagers have the wherewithal to spend countless dollars on advertising, on fancier packages, and of course, the brunt of this cost must be passed along to you, the consumer.

The private label packagers chant this song time and time again. So often has this been brought before the public, that the larger, better-known packagers hasten to point out that these manufacturers, screaming ceaselessly about "lower costs" are spending a like amount of money in packaging, advertising, etcetera, that the preaching is but a myth. They add too, that only the larger packagers can afford to do the research, to spend monies on testing, that you are — despite Governmental control and regulation — getting a better product when you pay more for it. They staunchly maintain that their own laboratories run tests that weigh far more heavily than the Government regulations do, that they package exceedingly pure, test with great care, and, they add, when you're taking medication to improve your health, you want to take the very best, and cost is not a factor.

Those are the arguments. Still, aspirin is aspirin, and as long as the dosage is the same, the healing of a headache will take place regardless of what brand of aspirin you take! Other factors do enter into this matter: if an aspirin is buffered to prevent stomach upset, we pay a bit more for the buffering. If the dosage is increased to provide more and faster relief, we pay extra for that. Check the grain content on the label, for obviously more aspirin in the tablet is going to cost more! When we take an aspirin to relieve a headache, we want the headache relieved as fast and as comfortably as possible. However, when you come up against a brand name and a private label that purport to do precisely the same thing for you, then you and you alone have to make the decision. In the final analysis, it's your problem that you're trying to cure, and it's your money that you're spending to cure it.

The fact of the matter is that some of the so-called "off-brands" have become as big and well known as the top brands, and the off-brands are now facing the selfsame problems that they created for the big names when they started. As in so many other fields, the wheel turns full circle!

How to take the medicine you buy is another matter that poses problems for many. The medicines that are to be taken orally usually come in the form of a pill, tablet, capsule or liquid. Sometimes the content of a single tablet is too strong, and the tablet may be scored for easy breaking. In most cases, simple pressure will cause the tablet to snap evenly into two parts, right along the score line. However, as dosages have a cumulative effect over a given period of time, do not be overly concerned if a small portion seemed to have parted over the score line onto the other side. A bit more or less will not usually harm you and is compensated for during the next dosage period by the remaining portion which makes up for it.

If the medication calls for "three times a day, with meals," try to understand that the label directions are simply attempting to make you take the medicine over a given time period. You are not supposed to take the medicine three times a day — with five minute intervals — but over the course of the day. As people usually have their meals some three or four hours apart, this is a convenient way to time your remedy and not forget to take it. Taking it with meals will separate the time that you take the medicine over a sufficient interval.

Should you take a medication before, during, or after a meal? This is another of those questions that plague physicians and pharmacists. If you have a stomach that is sensitive to the medication, you'll find that injesting the medicine after a meal allows it to set more easily than if you took the medication on an empty stomach. The results, of course, will be the same. The medicine will be absorbed into the system regardless of when you take it in relationship to the meal. Some medications interact badly with certain foods, and the label will so indicate.

Another serious area of concern is the business of dosage when it comes to liquid medications. One of the better-known cold remedies comes with a special cap that serves as a measuring cup as well. You fill the little plastic cup to the line and drink the stuff down. But if you check after you've quaffed the juice, you'll see a residual bit of the liquid sticking to the cup. Should that be inside you also? Or has the manufacturer allowed for this when he put the line into the cup? And if you *do* manage to get the last little bit by licking the cup, are you taking too much?

How about those directions that say "Take one teaspoonful." If you've had any experience with teaspoons at all, you *know* that no two are precisely the same. If you have a fairly large teaspoon, are you getting too much medication? And if your teaspoon is too small, are you getting sufficient?

The fact of the matter is that the liquid medications are extremely forgiving, and a bit more or less than called for will not harm you. Take a little too little, and all it means is that your condition may take longer to improve. Take too much and you may find a bit of stomach discomfort. There's no great danger either way, and we've known many people who carry a bottle of medication with them and simply swig a draught directly from the bottle, guessing at the dosage.

If you are concerned, by all means contact your local pharmacist, who can sell you a special measuring spoon for liquid medications. The bowl of the spoon is of plastic, is basically cylindrical in shape, and is fitted with an adjustable stop and barrier that can readily be aligned with demarcations in the spoon bowl as to quantities. Set the spoon, fill the bowl with the medication, then press the lever to expel the medication onto your tongue, where it is easy to injest.

People have some strange ideas about medications and dosages, and some of the ideas are potentially dangerous. "If this stuff was dangerous," they reason, "the Government wouldn't allow them to sell it." Nothing could be further from the truth. The dosages are clearly indicated on the label, and it's true that under ordinary circumstances there's little or no danger, provided that you cleave to the instructions on the bottle. Should you undertake to alter the instructions for whatever reason, you may be setting yourself up for problems. Yet people seem willing to run risks, taking too much too often.

Frequently people are not aware of the fact that certain medicines can interact badly with other medicines. Certainly any thinking user will observe labeled warnings and not take medicines in combination with others if the label warns against this. The reason is fairly obvious. Chemicals, whatever sort, can cause problems when injested in the wrong combinations, and if the label warns you against using medication "A" if you're already taking medication "B." With such an obvious warning, you should *not* take these in combination. In addition, when you are under a physician's care and taking a prescription drug that he recommends, you should check whether any of the available self-medicating remedies you are taking should be avoided. Ask your doctor? Certainly. His immediate concern is effecting your cure. He may easily overlook what seems in afterthought an important question. Naturally, since you're also concerned with your healing, you may also forget, but you can always call later and ask.

Medications For Children

Feeding medication to children is another area of great concern. Kids all know that medicines are supposed to taste bad, they may have difficulty in swallowing capsules or tablets, and getting a youngster to take his medicine can indeed be a problem.

You're surely going to find the so-called "flavored" medications, and while these may be a bit more palatable than the unflavored variety, the flavoring agents used often leave a great deal to be desired and present as great problems in feeding as the unflavored types do. They're *still* medicine, and you're still going to have problems in administering them.

Oddly enough, up to a certain point, youngsters seem to have no trouble in chewing and swallowing aspirin.

It's the recommendation of many physicians that you should not lie to the youngster, pretending that the medicine tastes good when it doesn't. By using such subterfuges you may get the first dose into your child, but you won't get another dose in, no matter what! Instead, explain that the stuff might not be the best tasting in the world, but that it is medicine and will make him or her feel better soon. You can offer a small treat after the dosing to take away the bad taste. Such honesty is usually rewarded by the child having more faith in you — and in the medication.

If the child has to take pills, tablets or capsules and has an aversion to taking these, there's still a way to get them down. Capsules usually can be opened by simply pulling the two halves apart. The medication inside can be spilled into a plain white paper that has first been folded in half and then opened. This will form a funnel-like trough, so that the powder can be then spilled into a spoon. This can than be mixed with water and given easily. Tablets can be ground to a powder as well. Place the tablet in the bowl of a large tablespoon, grind it to a powder with the heel of the bowl of a teaspoon.

With a bit of ingenuity, you can sometimes disguise a medicine in other foods that are more palatable. Try cutting a small pocket in a slice of bread, inserting the tablet in the pocket, then liberally coat the bread with jelly and offer it to the child. Chances are that the youngster won't even know he's taken the pill! With a bit of imagination, you can learn to conceal pills or capsules into various candies, cookies, or almost anything.

However, it's a good idea to inform your child after the entire course of treatment that he had the medication — even tell him how! Let him clearly understand that he has been cured of his illness *only* because he has had his medicine!

How Much To Take

Whether it's a child or an adult, keep in mind that prescription medicines should be taken until the entire dosage is completed. If the doctor prescribes twenty capsules, take all twenty, regardless of how much better you might feel after the first six or so. Complete the *entire* course of treatment! On the other hand, self-medications that are purchased without prescription may not require that you take a given amount during the course of treatment, but that you take them only until you're feeling better. This will mean that you may have additional of the nonprescription drugs after you're through taking them. With prescription medications, you won't have any left over, for unless the doctor instructs otherwise, you will use all of the medicine until it's gone.

Too often, druggists today type the scantest of information on your label for the prescription medication bottle. When you buy a nonprescription drug on the other hand, the manufacturers print all sorts of dosage information on the label and the package insert. It's up to you to read and follow these directions if you want the greatest benefit from the contents of the package. Because many of the packages are extremely small, you may have a bit of a problem reading the label directions which can be printed in miniscule type. The package insert will have far more room, and a larger type size can be used. It's our recommendation that the package insert be attached directly to the bottle with cellophane tape in such a way that when the insert is folded as it was when received, it will wrap easily and conveniently around the bottle or box, and an elastic band can hold it right there where it will not get lost.

Many people go a step further, too. They maintain a loose-leaf notebook in which package inserts and even bottle labels are kept. Whenever a new drug product is purchased, the information sheet is added to the file.

Be careful about dosages, for taking medications incorrectly can often result in more serious illness than caused you to take the medication in the first place!

The following material, reprinted from the Department of Health, Education, and Welfare, makes some interesting points that will surely prove of interest.

Medicines Without Prescriptions

No doubt you, like millions of other Americans, use nonprescription (or over-the-counter) drugs to get relief from minor problems such as headache, indigestion, constipation, mild aches and pains, and skin irritations.

There are thousands of over-the-counter (OTC) drugs most people can use safely and with beneficial results to relieve minor symptoms. Even though you can buy OTC drugs without a prescription, they should not be used all the time. OTC drugs should never be used regularly or over a long period. They can never "cure" disease, only relieve symptoms. If your problems persist, you should make an appointment to see a physician.

Before buying a drug product, you should read the label carefully to make sure the drug is the right one for the symptoms you have. And do not expect a "miracle cure." Sometimes advertising for over-the-counter drugs—on radio, television, or in newspapers — exaggerates the need for a drug, or creates a problem for you that does not even exist, or promises more results than you can expect. Advertising of OTC drugs is regulated by the Federal Trade Commission, which is taking action to see that drug advertising is honest and gives the product's risks as well as benefits.

As a consumer, you ought to view advertisements of OTC drugs carefully, and make sure you are not persuaded to buy something you don't need. No drug can make you look younger, lose weight, or even relieve a headache in an instant.

Your Physician and Pharmacist

Your physician and pharmacist are trained in drug therapy. They know what a drug is supposed to do and what adverse effects you can expect. They are good sources of information about drugs. Your pharmacist by law may not diagnose disease or prescribe a prescription medicine, but he may be able to help you. If your pharmacist recommends that your see a doctor, take his advice. If an adverse reaction to an OTC drug — or a prescription drug as well — is serious, consult your physician for advice.

The Importance of Labels

Federal law requires that the labeling of over-the-counter drugs must provide all the directions for use needed by the average person. This includes the conditions under which the drug should not be taken — for example, special instructions concerning its use (or nonuse) for infants, very young children, or the elderly. However, no amount of labeling is beneficial if you don't *read* the label and follow instructions. All the labeling on OTC drugs should be read and followed carefully — this may include the label on the package as well as a leaflet inserted in the package — and it is a good idea to check the label directions again, every time a medicine is used.

Adverse Reactions

Sometimes when you take an OTC drug you may have a side effect. That is, the drug may produce some effect other than its intended one. Sometimes these side effects are undesirable — they are then called adverse reactions. Whenever you have an adverse reaction, you ought to stop taking the drug right away. If an adverse reaction to an OTC drug is serious, consult your physician for advice.

It might be well to remember that you should *never use prescription drugs borrowed from someone else,* because of the danger of side effects or other complications. Also you should never use medicines that are old, since many drugs may become stale, or sometimes harmful or ineffective over long periods of time. At regular intervals, clear out your medicine cabinet and dispose of both prescription and OTC drugs that you have had on hand for a long time.

Safe Use of OTC Drugs

Used with care, over-the-counter drugs are safe for most people, and they serve an important function in overall health care. But there are dangers in overdoses; in combining drugs without your physician's advice; in using drugs incorrectly (because of not understanding your symptoms, or not following directions on the label); and in carelessness with drugs where children are concerned.

Use nonprescription drugs when you need to, but use them correctly — for temporary discomforts that do not require professional treatment.

Children and OTC Medicines

To make sure children are protected from accidental use of medicines or other products that could be harmful, the Poison Prevention Packaging Act requires that all such chemicals or drugs be enclosed in safety packaging. When you buy medicines, or other products that pose a potential hazard to children, look for safety packaging. In OTC drugs this means choosing a container with a top designed to be especially difficult for children to open or medicines encased in an individually wrapped package. Also it should be remembered that drug packages are designed especially for keeping the drugs placed in them safe and potent, so you should consult your pharmacist before transferring a drug to a different container or package. Buying safety-packaged drugs can be a tremendous help in preventing accidental injury to children — and perhaps even to careless adults. But don't think that safety packaging alone can protect children. You must remember to keep medicines and all other chemicals out of the reach of children, in locked cabinets, and to avoid taking medicines in front of children, or leading them to believe that medicine is candy.

What Do U.S.P. and N.F. Mean?

Very often you will see the letters U.S.P. and N.F. in in a drug you buy. U.S.P. stands for *United States Pharmacopeia,* N.F. stands for *National Formulary.* These are two independent organizations which set standards for the manufacture of drugs. Whenever a drug label has these letters on it, it means that the drug was made according to official standards, and you can buy and use it with confidence. This provides the consumer with additional assurance that OTC drugs are of the highest quality.

What is FDA* Doing?

FDA is responsible for assuring the safety, efficacy and proper labeling of all medicines. In 1972 FDA began a

*Food and Drug Administration

massive review of all medicines sold without prescriptions. When this study is complete, OTC drugs should be even safer and more effective than they are now, and labeling will be more uniform and clearer. FDA maintains constant vigilance over medicines sold in the United States. FDA inspects drug manufacturing plants, and also performs tests in its own laboratories, to make sure that all drugs are of the best quality.

If you ever buy an OTC drug — or any other product regulated by FDA, for that matter — which doesn't seem "right" and which may have been manufactured incorrectly, call the nearest FDA office. Look up the number in the phone book under United States Department of Health, Education, and Welfare.

The Dangers in Overdoses

OTC drugs that are safe in the dosage recommended on the label may be extremely dangerous in large overdoses. For example, aspirin is seldom thought of as dangerous, but there are numerous reports of accidental poisoning of young children who swallow too many for their young bodies to handle. In adults, excessive use of some pain-killing drugs may possibly cause severe kidney damage, and some drugs for relief of stomach upsets, when taken in excess, can cause an imbalance in the body's secretion of enzymes, perhaps resulting in serious digestive problems.

Overuse of other drugs, such as continued use of laxatives to relieve constipation, may only hide some underlying problem. You should never use any over-the-counter drug on a regular, continued basis, or in large quantities, except on your physician's advice. You could be suffering from a serious condition which requires professional medical treatment.

Using Several Medicines at the Same Time

Each drug (or medicine) you take not only acts on the body but may also alter the effect of any other drugs you are taking. Sometimes this can cause dangerous — even fatal — reactions. For example, aspirin increases the blood-thinning effect of medication prescribed for patients with heart disease. Therefore, a patient who has been taking such a medication may risk hemorrhage if he uses aspirin whenever he gets a headache. Before using any combination of drugs — prescription drugs with OTC drugs, or several OTC drugs together — it is important that you ask your doctor and follow his advice.

Drinking and Drugs

Alcohol may increase the effect of a drug. Sleeping pills and antihistamines are two types of drugs that interact with alcohol to produce drowsiness which may lead to injury. When taking either prescription or OTC drugs, you should ask your physician whether drinking alcoholic beverages could be dangerous in combination with the medicine.

Medicines and Drug Abuse

Experts believe there is a relationship between the abuse by adults of legitimate medicines, and the "drug culture" that has pervaded our country. You can do your share to reduce the likelihood that your children will become part of the "drug culture" by treating all medicines with respect, by letting your children know that medicines and drugs should not be used frivolously.

Chapter Five

Contraindications and Interactions

If there is one chapter in this book that is of tremendous importance — one chapter that should be considered "must" reading — it is this one, because it provides information that can save your life. By reading it, you will learn how to take drugs properly and safely.

And if there is one sentence in the entire book that could be called the most important, it is: Please read the labels. Read the labels, then read them again and understand them. Also read the box "stuffers" and package inserts that the manufacturer supplies. These are not simply advertisements — they tell you important, very important, things about the medications that you have purchased.

In this chapter, we're going to talk about contraindications and interactions, which are large words with even larger messages. What they mean is that under certain specified conditions and circumstances, these medications should not be taken.

Truth to tell, in most cases, your inspection and perusal of the listed contraindications will reveal no reason for you to not take the medicine. Still, it never hurts to examine these and play it safely. You might learn, for example, that the medication is contraindicated where other medications are being used. The medicines you are contemplating for example, might interact with the one you have been taking and the results could be sheer disaster! As a further example, you may find that if you are taking an aspirin-containing medicine and then take a second aspirin-containing medicine, the cumulative effect might cause you to overdose on the aspirin. Some medications can cause drowsiness, and the second medication, containing the same sleep-inducing drug could just knock you out. Other drugs cancel out the effects of the primarily taken drug, negating its value and worth.

Another type of contraindication is expressed in the label warning, "May cause drowsiness — not to be taken while operating machinery or automobiles." If you ignore the warning, the accident you have — or cause — will be entirely your own fault.

Allergic Reactions

Contraindications can bear on your own allergies, too. If your system is unable to tolerate certain drugs, you will manifest an allergic reaction in the form of rashes, or violent systemic upset. Surely, in this day and age of antibiotic treatments, you know if you are allergic to penicillin. You will know if you are allergic to eggs. Many vaccines are raised in egg cultures, and while the active ingredients might not hurt you, the base itself could cause damage. Sometimes, even if you know that you have an allergy, you might be tempted to ignore the consequences. A gentleman of our acquaintance is allergic to sheep's wool. So much so that during his military service in a cold climate he preferred to suffer the bitter cold rather than wear the warm woolen "long johns" that were issued. His first attempts to wear these resulted in constant itching and scratching. To this day, his clothing is all man-made fibers, and he shuns pure wool like the plague! Your author noticed that during a business meeting he spent much of the time scratching his head. We asked what sort of hair tonic he used, and he answered, rather suprised at the question. "Allergic to wool?" we asked. "Yes," he replied, "but how did you know?" Further investigation revealed that he was using a hair tonic with a lanolin base. Know what lanolin is made from? Sheep's wool. That's what!

Another common contraindication is against the use of alcoholic beverages while taking some medications. This too is fair warning. Often, you'll never know what hit you, or how you're liable to react.

It's not just the medications that contraindications can apply to, either. A youngster in a household ran out of toothpaste once, and arbitrarily used some of Grandma's. What he didn't realize is that Grandma had false teeth and her dentifrice was clearly labeled, "Not for use on natural teeth."

Knowing what contraindications and interactions are can protect you, obviously, but then it's up to you to relay the information to your family and thereby protect them.

Determining the correct dose is equally important. You must not simply assume that because you are big and bulky you ought to take a dose-and-a-half to make sure that there's enough of the stuff in your system. And maybe your boss does swallow aspirin like peanuts, and it doesn't seem to hurt him, but I'll bet he has an ulcer, too! Does this raise a cause-and-effect question in your mind? Play it safe and stick to label instructions. Of course, there are exceptions to every rule, and people have been known to take as many as 48 aspirins in a single day.

Charlie says you can take all the aspirin you want, as long as you take it with milk to "buffer" it. Let Charlie go that route. In fact, be a nice guy and *don't* let Charlie go that route! Warn him now.

When it comes to contraindications, especially with the patent or over-the-counter remedies, the only way to find out is to read the labels carefully.

Many of the packagers of these medications cannot be thought of as completely free of guilt, either. Frequently, they make claims in their advertising for their own products and at the same time make statements about competitive products. Faulty or falsified advertising, usually controlled by the FDA, can slip through, too. Innuendo is used, as is implication. The result can be a confusing maze for a gullible public. The campaigns presently being run for pain relievers is typical. "Don't trade your headache for an upset stomach!" warns one manufacturer, implying that his competitor's product will upset your stomach, but that his own will not. His competitor, on the other hand, makes a big thing about "fast relief" so that you will infer that his product provides faster relief than his competitor's! The nonaspirin pain relievers claim that their own products are best, and then compete with one another on the basis of price!

But back to contraindications.

What can you do if the medicine you want to use is contraindicated? You do not simply have to accept fate and suffer your illness to a natural conclusion. If you are unable to locate a suitable medication on your pharmacist's shelf, by all means consult with him. If you have a question regarding a nonprescription item, he or she has undergone training to prepare him exactly to answer your questions regarding such items, and his training continues long after he leaves school, reading the trade journals, the technical literature from manufacturers and the books available in the field to keep himself abreast of the latest developments.

There was a time when pharmacists were held in higher esteem. Money wasn't so easily available either, and before you went to a physician, you visited the local druggist. He wore a white coat, always had a friendly smile, and you called him "Doc." He could compound a prescription or a chocolate phosphate with equal skill. And nine times out of ten, good ol' Doc could tell you what was wrong and what you should take to fix it.

Today's pharmacist may not do as much basic compounding as he does counting out and packaging prepared capsules, pills and tablets. But don't underestimate this man's ability to advise you in the field he knows best.

Should a patent remedy be contraindicated, ask your pharmacist, and chances are that he'll be able to recommend something equally efficacious but without the contraindicated chemicals.

Implied, although not expressly stated under contraindications, is the matter of improper dosage. If you do not take a sufficient dose of the remedy, chances are that it will not do an appreciable amount of good. If you injest too much, it might very well harm you.

Dosage control is a difficult problem for the manufacturers and packagers of patent remedies, for it is a matter that is left entirely in the hands of the consumer. In the early days of medication, you usually bought a packet of folded papers in which the medication was folded into the individual sheets of paper. The medicine was in powdered form and you could pour the powder on your tongue and swallow it with a glass of water. Or you could dissolve the powder in the bowl of a spoon along with water, and take it that way. Seidlitz Powders, an effervescent laxative, are still sold in this form today.

Medications designed for oral ingestion are sold in the form of tablets, capsules, pills and liquids. Spansules, or timed-release medications, provide relief for up to 12 hours with a single dose. Liquid medicines used to be (and still are) listed with dosages in "teaspoonsful." Of course this is a fairly hit-or-miss system, as many teaspoons come in different capacities, but all-in-all, you can depend on getting approximately the correct dosage if you follow the label directions.

The packagers of liquid remedies have recently gone to the inclusion of a small plastic "shot glass" that measures precisely the amount of liquid you are supposed to take.

Many of the tablets are scored for easy breakage into two or four parts so that your dosage can be more easily regulated.

Children's medications are formulated with fruit flavor to make them more palatable. However, it has been our own experience in dealing with children that these so-called flavorings are usually either too weak or too intense, in either case, not contributing much in the way of taste.

Oddly enough, an adult cannot usually take a simple aspirin and chew it without grimacing at the strong, unpleasant taste! Kids, on the other hand, will chew and swallow an aspirin tablet without any qualms at all. But this is something they should not do.

Generally, taste is but a fleeting thing at best, and if a medication to be taken orally does have an unpleasant taste or aftertaste, this can usually be totally eliminated by following the medication with a strong citrus juice.

Other medications, such as eyedrops, are listed with dosages that recommend one or two drops in each eye. Don't be overly concerned if you should get three drops in one eye. The eye can only accept two drops, and any extra amount will simply run out of the eye.

Reactions

What few people realize about many medications is that they might have an allergic reaction to a given medication and should therefore find out from a physician about the same *family* of medications. Many medications are obtained from the same base. If your reaction is one to the base rather than to the active ingredient, any other medications that have been prepared in the same base will also cause a similar reaction!

This matter of reactions to certain drug products is a very individual thing, and it's just completely unsound to generalize. In most cases, you can depend on the drug product that you've been contemplating to be precisely what you expect it to be, to do exactly what you want it to do, and to be safe. There are exceptions, of course, but if you note any sort of adverse reaction, stop taking the medication at once and consult your physician.

In many instances, a reaction is not necessarily an allergic reaction. A friend of ours recently suffered severe stomach cramps after eating, and his concern was to get immediate relief. When he voiced his plight to the others, one offered an antacid tablet, another warned of the possibility of heart attack. They decided to try the antacid first, and if that offered no relief, they would get him to a physician. The symptoms of heart attack, as we have said, are often mistaken for the symptoms of gastric distress.

If the antacid had any effect at all, it was to make the pain even more severe. Our friend was rushed to the emergency room at a local hospital. He was given electrocardiogram tests which proved negative.

Subsequent examination revealed that he didn't have a hyperacidity problem — his case was just the reverse. It was a hyperalkaline problem which manifests itself in much the same way as hyperacidity! The antacid mint that he was given merely aggravated an already aggravated condition!

While the drug manufacturers take every possible precaution to avoid such problems, they cannot possibly anticipate everything that might happen. A good deal of the responsibility must devolve on you, and your best protection against difficulty is to read all of the available literature and act accordingly in your own best interest.

Yet what remains a constant source of amazement is that people — thinking, intelligent people — will time and again commit bonehead blunders that could as easily be avoided by simply familiarizing themselves with label instructions *before* taking medications!

It is extremely difficult to sympathize with somebody who, through his own neglect, brings compounded problems down on his head. The illogical reasoning that "if a patent medication was harmful, the Government would not let them sell it" is nonsensical. Yet many of the people who misuse and abuse such products react with just that question . . . "How come they can *sell* it?" People are always seeking out fall guys for their own mistakes, but rest assured that there's little consolation when you have made yourself even sicker to say that you didn't know, or that your pharmacist should never have sold you that stuff.

It's your job, your twofold job, to know what will go against your own particular grain, and then to read carefully stuffers and instructions to make sure that you do not buy or use anything that will not only be of no aid to you, but might even do you harm.

As we stated at the beginning of this chapter, it could be the most important chapter in the book. It can save you pain and agony, and maybe even save your life. Just remember to *caveat* the heck out of *emptor!*

How can you know? Short of a series of expensive and time-consuming tests, make a note of whatever reactions you might have to specific drugs and if you do have a bad reaction, don't take them again. Avoid any drugs in the same chemical family as well. And if you commence a course of treatment with any drug that gives you a bad reaction, stop taking it at once.

Side Effects

All medicines are double-edged swords. They can alleviate symptoms and in some cases cure disease. Hopefully, when you take a drug it will fulfill the primary function for which it was intended.

But some effects from medicines are not what you want. Medicines also cause undesirable or unexpected effects. These are known as "side effects," or adverse reactions, and can be caused by medicines bought with a doctor's prescription as well as medicines purchased over the counter.

You should be alert to the possibility that medications can cause side effects. You should also be aware that every medication has the potential to cause some unwanted effects in some people.

Unexpected or undesirable effects can be mild, such as a slight rash, mild headache, nausea or drowsiness. They can also be more severe, such as prolonged vomiting, bleeding, marked weakness or impaired vision or hearing. These symptoms are Nature's way of telling you that the medicine is acting adversely, and that you ought to do something about it.

One important fact that you ought to remember is that every individual reacts differently to medicines. Just because someone you know had no side effects from a drug, it doesn't mean you won't. For this reason, never take medication prescribed for someone else, even if you feel your symptoms are the same. And never give anyone else a medicine that has been prescribed for you. You may be doing a disservice by causing the other to have a bad reaction.

If a prescription drug you are taking causes an unexpected or undesirable effect, call your physician right away. He will know whether you should continue taking the medicine.

Often when your doctor is writing a prescription, he will tell you that it may cause some side effects. Listen carefully to what he says so you'll know what to expect. If you don't understand, ask your doctor to explain it again. It's important that you know just what to expect from the medicine before you take it.

If a side effect is unexpected or is unusually severe, your physician will have to make a decision. Should you continue taking the medicine because its desirable effects are so beneficial that they're worth the discomfort caused by side effects? Or should you stop taking the medicine?

You may not need to stop taking a prescription drug that has only mild side effects, but this decision is one you have to make with your doctor. Often he can prescribe another medicine that has fewer or less severe side effects but that can still help your condition.

If an unusual or undesirable reaction occurs from taking a medicine you bought over the counter without a doctor's prescription, you should stop taking it right away. Often the side effects known to occur from over-the-counter medicines are listed on the label. Read the label carefully before taking the medication. And if there are side effects, use common sense. If drowsiness may be expected, for example, you shouldn't drive or operate any machinery until the medicine's effect wears off.

Interactions

It's important to remember that mixing two types of medicines can often cause an unexpected and sometimes very severe reaction. You should never mix two medicines unless your doctor tells you it's all right. Alcoholic beverages are also drugs and shouldn't be mixed with medicines unless your doctor approves.

Your doctor and pharmacist are usually experts in the uses of medicines. They know what medicines should and shouldn't do. They are in the best position to answers any questions you may have when an unexpected reaction does occur.

Timothy J. Larkin is a special assistant to the Commissioner of Food and Drugs. In a recent issue of *FDA Consumer,* published by the Food & Drug Administration, he had the following comments regarding the mixing of medications. We felt that these were of sufficient importance to repeat them here.

> Although not the definition cited by scientists, chemistry could be defined as the science of combining substances so that the whole is usually surprisingly different from the sum of its parts. Take a positive ion of the soft metal sodium which can burn the skin or explode when mixed with water.

Combine this hazardous substance with a negative ion of the poisonous, greenish-yellow gas, chlorine. The result is not an even more dangerous chemical, but something quite different, the universal seasoning, the white currency with which Roman legionnaires were paid — salt.

Perhaps even more extraordinary is the end result of combining two atoms of hydrogen gas and one of oxygen. The product, water, possesses properties that would have been impossible to predict from the qualities of its constituents.

The results of some drug interactions are unimportant. Others, however, can mean the difference betwen successful and unsuccessful treatment; can produce a false reading of a laboratory test; can cause unexpected and possibly serious — even fatal — side effects; or can set off puzzling or misleading symptoms.

Although the FDA requires that the manufacturer of a new drug prove its safety and effectiveness, the drug producer does not routinely carry out, and is not required by law to carry out, tests for safety and effectiveness that involve simultaneous use of several drugs. One reason is that the whole problem of drug interactions is still new and incompletely understood. Another is that it is an endlessly complicated business.

Complicated, partially understood, but nonetheless important. Fortunately, largely due to the reporting of such interactions by physicians and pharmacists, a number of important facts have become known. As factual knowledge about potentially significant drug interactions emerges, the FDA requires that such information be reflected in the label that accompanies nonprescription (over-the-counter) medicines and the labeling information available to pharmacists and physicians for prescription drugs. FDA also publishes a widely distributed monthly collection of data about interactions and other important effects of drugs.

Drugs interact in a number of ways. One drug may make another act faster or slower, or more powerfully or less powerfully than it normally would. One drug may change the effect another drug has on the body.

A fairly common way one drug acts on another is by affecting the way it is absorbed, distributed, or broken down (metabolized) by the body. For example, let's assume that you are afflicted with a circulatory problem due to clotting of blood in an artery or vein. Your physician may prescribe an anticoagulant medicine — a medicine that "thins" the blood and thus helps dissolve the clot. If, at the same time, you are taking an antacid, even a nonprescription antacid, the anticoagulant may be absorbed at a slower rate than required to do its job properly.

Alcohol and anticoagulants can interact in two ways, both serious. Chronic alcohol abuse will speed up the rate by which the liver metabolizes or breaks down the anticoagulant, reducing its effect. But drinking a great deal of alcohol in a short period can slow down the metabolism. This can magnify the impact of the anticoagulant to the point where the blood becomes so thin it may be difficult to halt bleeding caused by an injury or from an ulcer aggravated by the alcohol.

Alcohol is a depressant like many drugs, such as tranquilizers and sleeping pills. It should be noted that a number of popular nonprescription cough and cold medicines contain up to 15 percent alcohol, and that alcohol interacts not only with anticoagulants but also with a number of other medicines. For example, if a person taking nitroglycerin for angina pectoris, a painful heart ailment, is also drinking alcoholic beverages, the result may be hypotension — low blood pressure — serious enough to cause a failure of the blood circulatory system.

In addition to interfering with absorption, distribution and metabolism, one drug can also either inhibit or hasten the excretion of another, and thus either exaggerate or reduce the effect of the drug. One common way this occurs is through the taking of nonprescription drugs that change the pH or acid level of the urine. Prescription medicines are formulated on the basis of a normal level of acid (pH) in the urine. But certain nonprescription drugs (such as those containing ammonium chloride, sodium bicarbonate, or citrates) change the pH, and this can interfere with the otherwise beneficial impact of the prescription medicine.

When a number of drugs are being taken, consideration must be given to the effect of adding one drug to another — their cumulative impact. This so-called additive reaction is especially important if the drugs are similar in their general effect.

There are some drugs which, when combined, produce reactions that go beyond what one might assume would result from adding the effect of one to the other. With such drugs, the end result is greater than the sum of the two parts.

Even commonly used nonprescription medicines can have potentiating effects. Aspirin greatly increases the blood-thinning effect of oral anticoagulants. Therefore, a person who is taking such medication may risk hemorrhage if he or she uses aspirin to alleviate a headache.

Many nonprescription cold remedies contain antihistamines which can produce potentiating effects when taken in conjunction with alcohol or with a wide variety of prescription and other nonprescription drugs, particularly those that act as central nervous system depressants, including anesthetics, barbiturates, hypnotics, sedatives and analgesics.

One important kind of drug reaction does not involve one drug interacting with another in the body to produce an unwanted side effect, but rather a drug that skews and confuses the results of diagnostic tests. Ordinary nonprescription drugs can have this skewing effect and so can vitamins. For example, laboratory tests to determine a patient's calcium or bone metabolism can be affected by excess use of laxatives. Vitamins A, D and K, as well as such common over-the-counter drugs as aspirin, can produce false positive or negative readings in a great number of important tests used by physicians to diagnose illness. And large doses of vitamin C can produce a false negative urinary glucose test which can, therefore, mask a diabetes condition.

How can you protect yourself against a harmful drug interaction? Here are some suggestions:

When your physician prescribes a drug for you make sure he knows what other drugs you are taking. All of them. Remember that the words "drug" and "medicine" mean the same thing, and that alcohol is a drug. Headache remedies, cold medicines, laxatives and other nonprescription medicines are drugs. When your physician asks, "Are you taking any other medicines?" no drug is too unimportant to mention. The drugs cited in this article are among the most widely prescribed medicines, but they represent only a few of the hundreds of drugs that involve significant interactions.

Don't start taking a second drug unless your physician knows about it. It's also a good idea to tell your pharmacist when he fills a prescription what other drugs you are taking. He may wish to set up a personal record so that he can tell at a glance if you may be exposed to a drug interaction.

Don't take a drug prescribed for someone else because it is "good for stomach pain," or whatever it is that is troubling you. The drug in that prescription may interact with something else you are taking, or it may not be suitable for you or your ailment.

Read the label. Over-the-counter medicines are required by FDA to contain information about significant drug interactions.

Remember that drugs have three names. There is the chemical name, which is usually not given on the label.

There is what is called the generic name, which is the official, established name for a drug; and there is the proprietary name or the trade-marked brand name for that drug.

It is important to remember this because the warnings printed on labels give the generic name. Thus, a number of nonprescription medicines such as the antacids warn against taking the medicine with tetracycline, which is the generic name of an antibiotic. However, Achromycin, Tetrex, Kesso-Tetra Syrup, Sumycin, Panmycin, Tetrocyn, and over a dozen others are proprietary names for tetracycline. So, unless you know the generic name as well as the proprietary name, you may be exposing yourself to a drug interaction. To avoid this, ask your physician or pharmacist to tell you the generic name of any prescription drugs you may be taking.

It is also worth remembering that numerous drugs contain more than one ingredient. Empirin, a medicine widely used for relief of simple headache and other discomforts, contains aspirin as well as phenacetin and caffeine.

Finally, since knowledge about drug interactions is by no means complete, and individuals differ in their reactions to drugs, you may possibly experience a reaction to a mixture of drugs that is unknown, not only to your physician and pharmacist, but to the medical profession generally. So, if you are taking more than one drug and you become ill, by all means report it to your physican or pharmacist.

Chapter Six

The Accessories

Before you can prescribe a nonprescription medication for yourself or your family, you'll have to make certain of exactly what your problem is. You're going to need certain accessories that can be kept handy in the medicine cabinet.

Probably the first of these will be a suitable thermometer. Either an oral or rectal type can be used, but you have to understand that these have different bulb endings and are not meant to be interchanged. The thermometer comes in a protective plastic case, and as a precision instrument, it should be handled with care. Before and after each use the thermometer should be wiped with alcohol, then shaken down so the mercury is all in the lower bulb, or at least well below the normal temperature readings.

To take body temperature, either insert the thermometer into the rectum (use a suitable lubricant, such as K-Y Jelly or petroleum jelly) and leave it in place for three minutes. The oral thermometer should be placed under the tongue, the lips closed, and held for a like period.

The front or reading surface of the column is a glass lens that is molded into place when the thermometer is made. By holding the tube horizontally and rotating it slightly, you can cause the mercury column to seem wider or narrower. Rotate the tube so the column is its widest, then read the figures inscribed on the face of the tube.

The electronic sciences have evolved an excellent solution to an old problem! There are now available and at exceedingly low prices (well under $15.00), electronic thermometers that read instantly. The wired probe is placed under the tongue, the "read" button is depressed, and you get an instant reading, either on a large meter-type dial, or an illuminated, digital display, your precise body temperature. One of the large advantages that this device offers is the reduction of the possibility of misreading the older, glass thermometer scale. There is also no need to wait the three minutes.

In addition to the thermometer, you're going to want a hot-water bottle, which is rubber with a waterproof seal at the top. To use this unit, unscrew the sealed cap, fill the bottle with extremely hot tap water, replace the cap, screwing it down tightly and then wrap the bottle in a thick towel to prevent burning the area to which it is to be applied. Check this constantly to see that the toweling has not worked loose, exposing the rubber surface. If the bag cools, refill it with hot water.

The cold ice bag is of similar construction, usually being a fabric-covered rubber-like material with a large screw-cap at the top. This is filled with ice cubes, the cap replaced, and the bag applied to the affected member. The ice bag is usually constructed with a pleated surface that allows it to remain where it is placed.

An enema bag is similar to the hot-water bottle, except that it is fitted with a molded-in portion at the bottom which permits it to be hung upside-down so that gravity will convey the contents of the bag through the rubber tube and out the molded end. The tube is fitted with a spring clamp that permits you to regulate the flow of the liquid.

There is also available a new form of enema that presents excellent convenience to the user, and indeed, many physicians carry these as part of the equipment in their "little black bags." These are one-time use enemas. They come boxed and in collapsible plastic bags. The box is opened, the sterile cover removed from the nozzle. The nozzle is then lubricated and inserted into the rectum. The bag is then collapsed, squeezing its liquid content into the lower tract where the relaxation can begin. The empty container is then disposed of.

Another device, considered an essential for feminine hygiene, is the douche. These once consisted of a red rubber bag suspended upside-down from a hook at the back of the bathroom door. A rubber hose with a spring stopper controlled the flow of the liquid into the vaginal area, and hard plastic inserts conducted the liquid into place. While these are still currently available, they are giving way to the one-time use douche, consisting of a collapsible bottle and a suitable screw-on tip. The douche is disposed of after a single use.

In Europe, the bidet (pronounced bi-day) is a necessary part of any bathroom. It is also used as a hygienic bath, and thanks to the popularity of foreign travel, many Americans came to know the value of this upward-spraying toilet-like contraption! The bidet is coming more and more into popularity in this country, and it provides a refreshing, cleansing bath.

A vaporizer is required, especially where young children are involved, and especially so if they are asthmatic. A physician might prescribe inhalants to be used with a device of this sort. It is plugged into a wall outlet, the necessary medication is inserted, and this is given off as a steam into the area surrounding the unit, so that the vapors can be inhaled into the lungs.

You might have to simply close the child's door and allow the vaporizer to expel its beneficial steam into the room. Where more concentrated inhalation is required, a large towel can be draped over the head and the vaporizer, thereby limiting the steam only to the air that is actually being inhaled.

Where dry heat must be applied for a protracted time period, the hot-water bottle is not suitable. In this situation a heating pad is called for. This is an electrical device that plugs into a wall outlet, usually has a heat control to regulate the amount it dissipates, and can easily be formed to or wrapped around the affected member.

One of the most frustrating situations one can face in an emergency is to apply a bandage and then not have scissors at hand with which to cut the bandage or adhesive tape. A blunt-end sharp pair of scissors is a real necessity. Having it in its proper place in the medicine cabinet and instructing family members that it is not to be used except for emergencies will ensure that it is always at hand when it is needed.

If certain family members have specific problems that might require specialized equipment on occasion, such equipment should be on hand and available. If a family member, for example, has a blood-pressure problem, a sphygmomanometer (blood pressure machine) should be on hand, along with a suitable stethoscope so that the pressure can be checked regularly. If somebody has a breathing problem that occasionally requires that oxygen be available, a small oxygen bottle should be kept on hand along with a proper mask and regulator. However, having the oxygen on hand is not sufficient. At least two family members should be well schooled in administering oxygen when it is needed.

Cotton swabs should be on hand, including the extra-long types used for the application of medication directly to the throat. Tongue depressors will also be needed. Both the swabs and the tongue depressors should be kept in sterile containers and sealed, and if you can obtain the tongue depressors in sanitary paper wrappings, so much the better.

When this chapter first went into preparation, we considered suggesting an assortment of ancillary first-aid materials, including splints, and a huge selection of assorted tapes and bandages. However, it soon became obvious that such things can easily be created when an emergency comes up. The emergency that requires such appurtenances will also require the services of a physician, and your time is usually better spent in transporting the patient to an emergency room at a nearby hospital, or getting a doctor to come and do what has to be done.

Antidotes for poisons are a necessity. Some poisons are not to be brought up, while others require an emetic. Carefully analyze the poisonous materials in your home and see to it — if you *must* have the poisons — that you also have suitable antidotes or emetics as needed.

Remember that only basic supplies will be needed. You're fitting out a home medicine cabinet, not a hospital operating room.

People today are very conscious of overweight, as well they should be. Surplus poundage is horribly debilitating, and the only way to reduce one's weight is by controlled diet and a well-thought-out program of controlled exercise to go along with it. One of the accessories that a dieter will want is a suitable bathroom scale.

How to Buy a Scale

There's scarcely a home that does not have a bathroom scale, and while this is all well and good, you may have noticed some slight discrepancy when you visited the doctor and found that his scale disagreed with yours. For most of us, this doesn't matter. All we really require at home is a relative indication of weight change, and the average bathroom scale is more than adequate to this task. However, there are differences in scales, and you should know about them.

The typical inexpensive bathroom scale is a lever-and-spring type, in which your weight on the platform is transmitted through a system of levers to a spring that is coupled to the indicator or dial. The scale is relatively accurate but is not legal for trade, nor can it be depended on for dead-accurate weight measurement. As long as you keep it on the same surface (not on a tile floor one day and a soft rug the next) it will provide a sufficiently accurate reading for normal home use. Do weigh yourself at the same time every day and in the same clothing. Your birthday suit will provide the most accurate readings.

The more accurate scales are the lever-and-beam scales such as your doctor uses. They maintain their accuracy over a long period by having a tare adjustment which enables you to reset the scale to zero before each use. Of course, these aren't very attractive, especially in a small bathroom. One scale company recently devised a smaller edition of this scale with a smaller beam height. It works the same way however and provides the same accuracy as the large medical scale. The only problem with these is that the beam oscillates until it settles, so you may have to wait a moment until the up-and-down bouncing comes to a rest. This type of scale may also be purchased from any medical supply company, which can be found by consulting the telephone classified directory.

A brand new version of the home medical scale is the digital readout scale, which is entirely electronic and operates from self-contained rechargeable batteries. It must be recharged after each 100 weighings. In this scale, an electronic stress cell is coupled between the read head and the platform levers. The resulting electronic signal is amplified and transmitted to the digital readout, which is dead accurate and illuminated.

Costs? The lever-and-spring bathroom scale can be had in a price beginning at about $8.00 and going up, depending on the "gingerbread." Get a scale with all sorts of fancy cork, leather or gilt, and the price rises. The mechanism inside remains the same. And incidentally, thanks to the pure physics of the matter, a square or rectangular platform will measure weight more accurately than the fancy flowered-shaped, round, or oval platforms. There's a more even weight distribution. If you're prepared to spend money in the order of $100 or more you can get the small lever-and-beam scale, a "scaled-down" version of your doctor's scale. And if you can go about $300, you can buy the cream of the crop, the new digital readout scale.

Check your own weight before buying any scale. Bathroom scales usually measure up to somewhere around 300 pounds. If you weigh 350 pounds (and many people do!) the bathroom scale will be useless to you.

Make certain, too, that you can read your scale. See that the numbers are large enough so you can look down from your own height and read them. Make sure, also (and this might sound funny, but can be a problem for some) when you are on the scale, that your stomach does not protrude to a point where you are unable to see the numbers. The scale that you cannot read is utterly useless.

Chapter Seven

Analgesics

If there is one most common nonprescription drug item that everyone seems to know about and use regularly, it has to be aspirin. It puts us in mind of the chap who went to the pharmacy and asked the druggist for a bottle of acetylsalicylic acid tablets. "Do you mean aspirin?" asked the druggist. "Funny," the man said, "I can never remember that word!" But pain isn't funny. Not when you're affected by it, and despite Imogene Coca's famous comment that "A little pain never hurt anybody," we fail to see anything to recommend pain.

Of course, pain can be treated with self-medications, but if the symptoms persist for more than ten days, proper advice should be sought. Any recurring or continuous condition must be brought to a physician's attention. Pain is the body's way of informing us that something is wrong. If you take a pain reliever to mask the pain, seeking immediate relief, you are disguising a symptom — not correcting the condition. Only your physician can recognize and help correct what might be a serious problem.

People who have frequent pain can ask their family physicians for a prescription drug that will act more rapidly than any nonprescription drug available. The physician, acting on his own knowledge of the individual's emotional stability and common sense, can prescribe such drugs in limited amounts.

Many definitions of pain have been formed, and there is not the least doubt that everyone has experienced it. Beecher, a recognized authority on the subject, defines pain as follows:

> Unfortunately, pain is a universal experience of mankind and everybody knows what is meant by it; so this discussion will concern itself only briefly with past unsatisfactory attempts to define pain. Pain is, it must be admitted, uncommonly difficult to define. But attempts at definition are useful in that they throw light on the process and on the nature of the difficulties encountered.
>
> Pain is a subjective matter clearly "known to us by experience and described by illustration." There seems little point for the present purposes to labor a definition of what all understand. Lexicographers, philosophers, and scientists have none of them succeeded in defining pain. Having said that it is the opposite of pleasure, or that it is different from other sensations (touch, pressure, heat, cold) or how it is mediated (through separate nerve structures), or what the kinds of it are (bright, dull, aching, pricking, cutting, burning), or what kinds of things will produce it (trauma to nerve endings, or to nerves, electric shocks, intense stimulation of the sensations of touch, pressure, heat, cold), or what it comes from (injury, bodily derangements, or disease), or that certain types of mild stimulation can probably be stepped up to a painful level through conditioning or what some reaction patterns to it are (escape or avoidance), none of these individual statements, nor indeed their sum total, provides a definition of pain.

Over-the-counter analgesics are both safe and effective for the treatment of the symptoms of minor aches and pains. Minor pain, for the purposes of self-medication, can be described as pain that is self-limited and which requires no special treatment or prior diagnosis by a doctor. The pain is usually described as being of mild to moderate intensity as opposed to sharp, severe or protracted pain. Even though no medical treatment is required for minor aches and pains, analgesics may be desirable to reduce their intensity and provide relief and comfort to the sufferer. People who have to work or maintain normal daily activities, or those who seek comfort in their homes, may find these agents particularly useful.

Usually you'll find the words "For the temporary relief of occasional minor aches and pains" on the labels of all over-the-counter analgesics. The word "occasional" is included, because recurrent, chronic or persistent pain might require a physician's diagnosis of its cause. For example, frequent headaches, joint pain or lower back pain which flares up periodically may indicate pathologic conditions that should not be treated with over-the-counter medications except under the advice and supervision of a physician. Regardless of the type of pain, these agents should not be used in adults for more than ten days. If symptoms persist beyond this period, become more severe, or if new ones occur, you should see a physician at once. In children under twelve years of age, this time period should be reduced to five days.

How do Analgesics Work?

Analgesics alleviate pain principally by a peripheral effect rather than by a central effect. The best available evidence for this is based on the studies of Lim, who, in 1967, induced experimental pain in animals and human volunteers, and demonstrated that the actions of aspirin and acetaminophen were predominantly on the peripheral nervous system and not on the brain.

In addition, there is evidence that a portion of the pain relief provided by analgesics that also have anti-inflammatory activity is due to a peripheral effect of decreasing the inflammation which removes one source of stimulation of pain receptors. The basic mechanisms of the action of the analgesics as far as inflammation reduction does not extend to the acetaminophen types.

Fever

The ordinary individual has a normal body temperature of 98.6°F (37°C) taken orally. The rectal temperature is 99.6; axillary temperature is 97.6. Although most individuals have an 0.5°C variation during a 24-hour period, or over several days, this is still considered to be within the normal range. Fever can be defined as a body temperature above the normal, and it may or may not be accompanied by pain.

Attitudes toward the presence of fever have undergone a change over the years. Fifty years ago, the reduction of fever was an end to be attained for its own sake. Today, fever is recognized as a symptom of disease, rather than a disease itself. Once the cause of the fever is ascertained, that cause is treated and the treatment of fever *per se* becomes secondary to removal of the underlying cause.

The causative agents of fever are referred to as pyrogens. These may be differentiated into two basic categories: those pyrogenic agents which are external to the body, such as those produced by infectious agents and referred to as exogenous pyrogens, and those pyrogenous substances which are produced by the body, referred to as endogenous pryogens. It is now generally accepted that the cells capable of producing endogenous pyrogens are activated by either exogenous pyrogens or endogenous factors. Those endogenous factors include inflammation, tissue damage, etc., which release endogenous pyrogens, and it is this circulating material which is the common mediator of fever.

An area at the base of the brain plays a primary role in the regulation of body temperature. In fever the balance between heat production and heat loss is still regulated by the hypothalamus, but this sets the body temperature at a higher than normal level. Fever can be reduced by the administration of antipyretic drugs. The antipyretics are said to act to "reset" the "thermostat" so that the body temperature will decrease toward normal. Heat production is not changed, but blood flow and sweating control heat loss. The perspiration is not due to a direct effect of the antipyretics on peripheral blood flow or the sweating mechanism, but rather to a central action on the hypothalamus.

It must be remembered that fever can be symptomatic of a serious illness, and that its cause, when not known, should be determined immediately, especially if it is marked (over 103°F), persists over 72 hours or recurs. However, when fever is due to the common cold or flu, it may be safely reduced by the administration of antipyretics. Analgesics such as salicylates or acetaminophen (Tylenol and Datril are examples) are good antipyretics. You'll find the words "For the reduction of fever" on the labels.

Inflammation

Inflammation and many rheumatic diseases are usually accompanied by pain and sometimes fever. In many rheumatic conditions the object of the therapy is to stop the disease process. This usually requires doses of drugs higher than those recommended for home remedy use. Furthermore, symptomatic self-medication with relief of accompanying pain may still allow permanent degenerative processes to continue. In certain inflammatory conditions, the inflammation is due to infection — in which case specific antibiotic therapy will be indicated. That is, inflammation of the joint or skin is due to a bacterial infection, and if antibiotics are not provided early in the course of the disease, infection of the bloodstream or spread of infection may occur. It is therefore concluded that over-the-counter drugs for the treatment of inflammatory conditions and rheumatic diseases should be used only under the advice and supervision of a physician.

Headache

It seems that whatever field of endeavor you're in, sooner or later, you're going to get a headache just by working at it. Unlike upset stomach, headache is not caused by what you eat as much as by what "eats" you! Headache is about as unpleasant a condition as you can develop, and because it is usually caused by stress, it reduces you to a point where you cannot continue to work. If your work is giving you a headache, the headache makes you stop working. It's nature's way of controlling the stress that induced the headache in the first instance.

But we are a nation of pill poppers, taking analgesics for the relief of headache pain so that despite nature's warning, we can continue to work. A brief survey of the numerous over-the-counter analgesics will reveal the extensive use of claims for "headache," "simple headache," "common headache" or "occasional headache." Many combination products contain additional nonanalgesic ingredients for such specifics as "sinus headache" or "nervous tension headache." Regardless of the descriptive terminology, "headache" is a very common term for a pain that affects almost everybody at one time or another.

Headache is a unique symptom. Unfortunately, it is an ambiguous term for pain having many different etiologies which can originate in almost any part of the body. Most headaches are transient, usually lasting less than one day. Some types of headache are chronic and may recur over a period of months or even years. The so-called "occasional headache" may be secondary to many other factors, including fatigue, tension, eyestrain, fever or even alcohol injestion. The chronic or recurrent headaches may be caused by more serious underlying diseases such as vascular disturbances, brain tumor or abcess, intracranial lesions or lesions of the eye, ear, nose or throat.

Vascular Headaches

A common feature of all vascular headaches is physiological changes in cranial blood vessels. In a majority of cases there is a tendency for these vessels to become distended. The vessel walls are then less able to accommodate changes in blood pressure, resulting in a more direct transmission of pressure variation to sensory receptors in the brain, which are interpreted as pain.

One type of vascular headache, the hypertensive headache, is related to elevation in the systemic arterial blood pressure. Another type of vascular headache is the common migraine. It has been estimated that nearly 12 million people in the United States suffer from migraine, and 8 percent of all headaches seen by the physician are attributable to migraine. A common feature of the migraine headache is a recurrent, throbbing, unilateral head pain. OTC analgesics are usually not appropriate for the treatment of hypertensive or migraine headaches, which require diagnosis of the disease by a physician and usually treatment with drugs available only by prescription.

Next to migraine, the most common vascular headache is the toxic vascular headache produced by fever, for which OTC analgesics may be indicated. It has even been suggested that alcohol can produce a toxic vascular headache commonly referred to as a hangover headache. Another form of toxic vascular headache which is common among heavy coffee drinkers occurs after withdrawal of caffeine.

Psychogenic Headaches

The second major type of headache, the psychogenic headache is one of the most common, accounting for up to 90 percent of the chronic headaches seen by a physician. The terms "muscle contraction" and "tension" headaches have been used synonymously for this condition for almost 40 years. These headaches are not vascular in nature or associated with traction or inflammation. Various factors which may cause a psychogenic headache include the individual's marital relations, occupation, social relationships, life stresses and habits. Apprehension, anxiety, posttraumatic experiences and depression can precipitate the symptoms. This form of headache is usually accompanied by persistent contraction of the muscles of the head, neck and face. The headache is diffuse in nature and the symptoms are usually described as a generalized pain not localized on one side of the head. In some individuals, it is described as a sense of pressure rather than a true pain.

Since psychogenic headache symptoms may be relieved by opiates or barbituates but not usually by analgesics, OTC analgesics are not recommended.

Treating Occasional Headaches

The occasional headache is self-limited and requires no definitive medical treatment. However, the over-the-counter analgesics are useful for symptomatic treatment. For example, in many situations, an OTC drug may be desirable to reduce the intensity and duration of the headache, providing relief to the sufferer and enabling him to return more readily to normal activity. As in adults, the use of suitable OTC analgesics in properly administered doses are effective for children. However, the treatment of the psychogenic headache caused by stress situations at school or disturbed family relationships at home should stress counseling rather than the use of drugs.

Labeling claims for analgesics are limited to the statement "For the temporary relief of occasional minor pains, aches and headache." The term "headache" is an acceptable labeling claim because of the wide acceptance and usage of over-the-counter analgesics by the general population for headaches as caused by muscle fatigue from occasional overexertion, for example, as opposed to the more complex migraine headache. It is believed that the consumer can usually distinguish the symptoms of this form of headache, which can be suitably relieved by self-medication with an appropriate OTC analgesic, from other forms of headache or pain requiring the attention of of a physician.

Mucosal Erosion of the Mouth

The previously discussed analgesics are systemic types, in that they must be fully injested in order to function. They are not topical analgesics. We have heard of people with toothache, for example, placing an aspirin tablet in the cheek against the offending tooth in the hope that the dissolving aspirin will more rapidly work to allay the pain. This is totally unfounded, for the aspirin must dissolve and be swallowed before it can work. By the same token, dissolving an aspirin and swallowing it so the liquid can "wash" over a sore throat will do not the least bit of good until the aspirin reaches the stomach where it can be transmitted through the system.

Aspirin-containing gum can produce a severe lesion of the inner wall of the cheek, which will heal only upon discontinuation. Aspirin tablets applied directly to the mucous membranes of the mouth for local anesthetic effect have resulted in oral lesions on the roof of the mouth. Aspirin tablets allowed to remain in contact with mucous membranes of the mouth for 30 minutes produced a white opaque mucous membrane capable of being peeled off with the slightest manipulation.

In tests, a quarter of several commercial plain, buffered, and combination aspirin tablets were placed between the lower lip or cheek and gums of several subjects for 30 to 60 minutes. In every case, the aspirin produced an irregular opaque lesion with the sloughing of dead cells characteristic of acute necrosis.

Warnings

Aspirin is ordinarily considered a fairly mild, harmless analgesic. However, aspirin poisoning due to overdose can be severely harmful, even fatal. Restrict your intake to recommended doses and do not exceed these. It should also be pointed out that people suffering certain inflammatory joint disturbances are given massive doses of aspirin products far in excess of recommended dosages, but this can be done only under a physician's care. The usual warning is to watch for a ringing in the ears, which serves as an indication of overdose. Be on guard against the same symptoms yourself.

RECOMMENDED ADULT DOSAGE SCHEDULES FOR STANDARD AND NONSTANDARD ASPIRIN, ACETAMINOPHEN OR SODIUM SALICYLATE DOSAGE UNITS

Dosage unit[1] (mg (gr))	Initial dosage units[2] (mg)	Frequency[3] (tablets/hours)	Dosage units/day[4] (tablets (mg))
Standard dosage schedule			
325 (5)	2	2 after 4	12 (3,900)
Nonstandard dosage schedule			
325 (5)	2 to 3 (650 to 975)	2 after 4	12 (3,900)
400 (6.15)[5]	1 to 2 (400 to 800)	1 after 3	9 (3,600)
421 (6.48)[5]	1 to 2 (421 to 842)	1 after 3	9 (3,789)
485 (7.46)[5]	1 to 2 (485 to 970)	1 after 4 or 2 after 6	8 (3,880) 8 (3,880)
500 (7.69)	1 to 2 (500 to 1,000)	1 after 3 or 2 after 6	8 (4,000) 8 (4,000)
650 (10)[5]	1 (650)	1 after 4	6 (3,900)

[1]The amount of drug contained in a single dosage unit.
[2]The maximum number of dosage units that cannot be exceeded when dosing is initiated.
[3]The number of dosage units per time interval.
[4]The maximum total number of dosage units that cannot be exceeded in 24 hours regardless of the initial number of dosage units taken or the frequency of repeated dosing.
[5]This nonstandard dosage schedule does not apply to acetaminophen since only the 500 mg (7.69 gr) nonstandard dosage unit is recognized by the Panel.

INTERNAL ANALGESICS

Product (Manufacturer)	Aspirin	Phenacetin	Salicylamide	Acetaminophen	Caffeine	Other
Alka-Seltzer Pain Reliever/ Antacid (Miles)	324mg					sodium bicarbonate, 1.904g Citric Acid, 1.0g
Anacin (Whitehall)	400mg				32.5mg	
Arthritis Pain Formula (APF) (Whitehall)	486mg (Micronized)					aluminum hydroxide, magnesium hydroxide
Bayer Aspirin (Glenbrook)	324mg					
Bayer Children's Aspirin (Glenbrook)	81mg					
Bayer Timed-Release Aspirin (Glenbrook)	650mg					
Bromo-Seltzer (Warner-Lambert) (Granules)		130mg/capful		325mg/capful	32.5mg/capful	sodium bicarbonate and Citric Acid to yield 2.8gm citrate/capful
Buffaprin (Buffington)	324mg					magnesium carbonate 97.2mg aluminum glycinate 48.6mg

Empirin Compound (Burroughs-Wellcome)	227mg	162mg		32mg	
Excedrin (Bristol-Myers)	194.4mg		129.6mg	97mg	64.8mg
Excedrin P.M. (Bristol-Myers)	194.4mg		129.6mg	162mg	methapyrilene fumerate 25mg
Liquiprin suspension (Norcliff-Thayer)				60mg/1.25ml	
Sine-Aid (Johnson & Johnson)	325mg				phenylpropanolamine hydrochloride, 25mg
St. Joseph Aspirin (Plough)	325mg				
St. Joseph Aspirin for Children (Plough) (Chewable)	81mg				
Tylenol Extra-Strength (McNeil)				500mg	
Vanquish Caplet (Glenbrook)	227mg			194mg	33mg	magnesium hydroxide, 50mg aluminum hydroxide gel, dried, 25mg

Chapter Eight

Vitamins

To some people, vitamins seem at first blush to be the ultimate treatment for any or all bodily ills. They can be taken on a regular basis, seem safe enough, since the body may only absorb the quantity of those vitamins that it requires and will possibly expel the rest. There seems to be some dichotomy here, however, for there have been cases of vitamin poisoning brought on by overdose.

In most cases, the Government specifies the MDR, or Minimum Adult Daily Requirement, of each of these vitamins. Some relatively new vitamins have not had an MDR established as yet. Vitamin E is typical of this, and yet you can purchase it in capsules ranging from 20 to 1,000 milligrams.

The proper way to take vitamins is by eating a healthy, well-balanced diet. If you do, vitamin supplements will be unneccessary. However, few of us eat that properly or well, so we supplement with multiple vitamins, taking these on a daily basis.

When special or specific problems occur, we tend to take massive doses of those vitamins that may have a beneficial effect. Nobody knows what will cure the common cold, but many people take massive doses of vitamin C to offset the problems.

Multivitamins are easily and readily available, but these supply only the minimum adult requirement and, to be effective, must be taken on a regular and ongoing basis. Should you have a specific vitamin deficiency, your physician alone should decide this and recommend a vitamin supplement for you. While you can easily purchase vitamins over the counter, you are hardly qualified to make the decision by yourself as to what needs you may have or how much you should take.

Vitamins are not always taken internally. We have learned that a lot of people are using vitamin E externally. Should they notice a sore, a growth or other form of skin problem — even minor cuts and bruises — they take a vitamin E capsule, pierce it with a pin, and squeeze the oil-like fluid over the spot to promote healing. The method is used on any skin outbreak, including rashes, cuts and wounds; the irony of it is that it often seems to work! The Government doesn't comment on this, for there is not yet sufficient information.

When it was first introduced, vitamin E was said to have amazing restorative powers, especially in the area of sexual potency. The claims were more implied than actually made, and because sexual responsiveness is so subjective a function, it is difficult to pinpoint any facts that can indicate a yes-or-no documentation.

Sexual responsiveness is an important thing to many people. You can depend on it if you have a new product that you'd like to introduce, simply claiming sexual powers for it will make your fortune.

One such product currently offered is based on ancient oriental belief. You can now buy Korean Ginseng, purified, pulverized and bottled in tablets or capsules. Rhinocerous horn is still another specific for this problem.

Vitamins are not of the same category. Vitamins, properly taken and properly prescribed, can have excellent and beneficial effect. But you have to know what you are taking, why you are taking it, and how much you need. Only your own family physician can tell you these things.

Despite the fact that the vitamins are on prominent display and that you can buy them easily and with no control, keep in mind that they are not the universal cure-all, the panacea for all ills of mankind. Sometimes they can do more harm than good.

Product (Manufacturer)	Vitamin A IU	D (IU)	E (IU)	Ascorbic Acid (C) mg	Thiamine (B1) mg	Riboflavin (B2) mg	Niacin mg	Pyridoxine Hydrochloride (B6) mg
B-Complex Caps (North American)				300	1.5	2.0	10	0.1
B-Complex Tabs (Squibb)					0.64	0.66	8.1	0.9
Brewer's Yeast (North American)					0.06	0.02	0.15	0.007
Chocks (Miles)	5000	400	15	60	1.5	1.7	20	2.0
Feminaid (Nion)	5000	400	10	200	2.0	3.0	15	25
Femiron with Vitamins (J. B. Williams)	5000	400	15	60	1.5	1.7	20	2.0
Flintstones (Miles)	5000	400		60	1.5	1.7	20	2.0

Geritol Liquid (per 5ml) (J. B. Williams)					5.0	5.0	100	1.0
Monster Vitamins (Bristol-Myers)	3500	400		60	0.8	1.3	14	1.0
Multiple Vitamins (North American)	5000	400		50	3.0	2.5	20	1.0
Myadec Tabs and Caps (Parke-Davis)	10,000	400	30	250	10.0	10.0	100	5.0
One-A-Day (Miles)	5000	400	15	60	1.5	1.7	20	2.0
Poly-Vi-Sol (Mead Johnson)	2500	400	15	60	1.05	1.2	13.5	1.05
Stresstabs 600 (Lederle)			30	600	15.0	15.0	100	5.0
Theragran (Squibb)	10,000	400	15	200	10.0	10.0	100	5.0
Unicap (Upjohn)	5000	400	5	45	2.8	3.2	36	

Product (Manufacturer)	Cyanocobalamin (B12) micrograms	Folic Acid micrograms	Pantothenic acid, mg	Iron mg	Calcium mg	Phosphorous mg	Magnesium mg	Other
B-Complex Caps (North American)			1.0					dried yeast, 100 mg dessicated liver 70 mg
B-Complex Tabs (Squibb)	1.0							
Brewer's Yeast (North American)			0.05					
Chocks (Miles)	6.0	400						
Feminaid (Nion)	10.0	100	10.0	18	126			zinc, 10 mg potassium, 10 mg
Femiron with Vitamins (J. B. Williams)	5.0	100	10	20				
Flinstones (Miles)	6.0	400						

Geritol Liquid (per 5ml) (J. B. Williams)	3.0		4.0	15			methionine, 100 mg choline bitartrate, 100 mg
Monster Vitamins (Bristol-Myers)	2.5	50	5.0				
Multiple Vitamins (North American)	1.0		1.0				
Myadec Tabs and Caps (Parke-Davis)	5.0			20		25	copper 2 mg, zinc 1.5 mg manganese 1 mg iodine 150 micrograms
One-A-Day (Miles)	6.0	400					
Poly-Vi-Sol (Mead Johnson)	4.5	300					
Stresstabs 600 (Lederle)	12		20				
Theragran (Squibb)	5		20				
Unicap (Upjohn)							

Chapter Nine

First Aid

When a major first aid emergency occurs, the first step is, of course, to phone the doctor or emergency squad. Any first aid given should be in the nature of emergency treatment until the doctor (or other help) arrives. Deep wounds need immediate and expert trained medical attention. But as we all know, not every emergency calling for first aid treatment requires a doctor's care.

We must point out at the very outset that this chapter will *not* be simply an emergency, hurry-up course in first aid. There are more than ample materials available for the reader who desires to explore this in further detail. Rather, this chapter will discuss those materials and medications that are used in first aid treatment around the home and will detail the products necessary to the proper administration of first aid.

People *are* going to hurt themselves or have other medical emergencies. The contents of the medicine cabinet that are devoted to first aid needs are, for the most part, for the purpose of preventing infection and relieving pain. However, pain is an indication that something is wrong. To relieve the pain and having done so reach the decision that further medical attention is not required is a gross error. Anything beyond the simplest cut or scrape severe enough to require treatment is sufficiently serious to warrant medical attention.

What should be on hand for first aid depends on your own needs, of course, but make certain that you have adequate quantities of materials for caring for punctures, impacts, burns and scalds, as well as scrapes and bruises.

Children are forever coming in with minor scrapes and scratches that can easily be treated at home. When you apply such treatment, it is a wise idea to keep track of the treated area, and if it seems to become infected or puffy, consult a doctor at once.

The minor wound, the result of a small scratch, should first be thoroughly cleansed, and your best ally in this is ordinary soap and water. We're talking here about skin-surface cuts, not the severe kind that sever veins or arteries. Cleaning the surface of the wound will remove most of the blood, a cause for fear in itself. With the wound cleansed, an antiseptic should be applied, and this is your next big decision — what kind of antiseptic should be used?

In the old days, you had a choice of Mercurochrome, tincture of iodine or hydrogen peroxide. Today we have even wider choices. The most popular antiseptic today, and perhaps one of the best, is tincture of Merthiolate. This of course comes along with a sting that will make anybody howl. Milder antiseptics such as Bactine do as good a job, but with a great deal less pain.

What we cannot overstress is that any wound which breaks the skin can result in problems that go far beyond the healing of the wound itself. Tetanus is but one of the problems that can result from a puncture wound, and there are many, many others that you must and should be aware of, including a vast array of infections.

There's another thing you should know as well. When a wound occurs, there are pain and fear to contend with in addition to the wound. It may seem out of place in a book like this, but a little "mother hen" treatment surely helps to heal some of the side effects, if not the wound itself. It doesn't take much effort to cluck over somebody that's hurt and offer a little kindness and sympathy.

Your best ally as a first step is ordinary soap and water. If you can, begin by cleansing the wound and the field, the area around the wound, with a good washing in soap and water to remove any dirt that may have lodged in the wound. Work up a good, sudsy lather, and then after this has been done, flood the area with clear running water.

What do you require in the way of medicines for first aid? For cuts and bruises you're going to want an antiseptic cleansing agent first. It won't hurt to have a medium-size bottle of hydrogen peroxide on hand to help flush the wound and clean it.

Now you'll want to apply a good antiseptic. The wound should then be covered to help prevent infection. For this you should have on hand an assortment of bandages, and we recommend the one-inch and two-inch sizes just for starters. For larger needs, get a packet of three- and four-inch sterile gauze pads. To hold these in place on the wound, you'll want some surgical adhesive tape, and we suggest the half-inch width as a good all-round answer. Keep in mind that the adhesive will have to be removed one day, and always wrap first with a bandage and then apply the tape. If the tape does not touch the skin directly, there's no problem in removing it. You simply avoid the painful problem of stripping the tape from the skin — an especially hairy problem if the subject has a hairy skin and a low threshold of pain.

How you go about handling bandages is also important. Too often we've seen people take the simple adhesive bandage from its sanitary wrapper, pull away the plastic strips that protect the adhesive and then actually handle the sterile gauze itself before applying it to the wound.

For smaller wounds we recommend the self-adhesive bandage which comes in assorted shapes and sizes to suit almost any need. Again, we suggest the type with a treated pad that will not cling to the skin, the sores or a healing scab.

Some puncture wounds result in the item which caused the puncture remaining behind in the skin. Before treatment is completed, you must remove the item that caused the puncture. Splinters and slivers must be removed, or the wound may heal and close over the foreign object, leaving the path open for later infection. Also, if the foreign body is not removed, the wound may not heal at all, and infection and festering is the result. You should have a good pair of surgical tweezers for such jobs, not the usual run of cosmetic tweezers. If you can, get a tweezer with a built-in magnifier attached. Remember, however, that you are not a surgeon, and if you are unable to quickly and easily remove the offending object, consult with a physician who can.

You're going to want a box of sterile cotton swabs. These are essential to the removal of foreign objects in the eye. Usually, such objects are found not clinging to the orb of the eye, but rather to the underside of the eyelid. To effect such removal, place a small matchstick over the eyelid, then fold the lid over the matchstick. In most instances, the foreign body can then be gently lifted away with the swab. If the object cannot be located or is difficult to remove, immediately stop your efforts and consult a physician. In some cases, you may learn that this is not a foreign object at all, but the start of an infection that should have immediate medical attention.

Almost a necessity, too, is a device that appears to have fallen into disuse. But you can still obtain a bottle of eyewash with an eyecup attached to the cap. If the eyes are simply tired, the eyewash provides an excellent relief. Simply fill the cup with liquid, hold the cup to the opened eye, then tilt the head all the way back, flushing the entire orb with the liquid.

For a quicker form of relief, there are eyedrops that can be used, and these require only that the head be tilted back, two or three drops applied into each eye, and then that the eye be moved rapidly back and forth, up and down to cover the entire eye with the fluid. The drops come in small, convenient bottles that are easy to carry with you and use wherever and whenever the need arises.

Another convenient product in the form of drops is used to dissolve collected wax in the ears. This is far safer than probing into the ear with anything from hairpins to paper clips, as many people do. One of our advisory board even claims that the only thing you should ever put into your ear is an elbow, and your OWN elbow, at that! More ear damage is done by such probing than can be imagined, and the ear-wax drops are a far safer method.

Another emergency that frequently requires attention around the home is burns and scalds. There are many old wives' tales regarding suitable treatment for such problems, the most popular being that butter should be applied. The fact of the matter is that almost *anything* that covers the burned area will provide relief from the pain. Plunging the affected area into water is the best procedure. Use the medication designed and meant for such accidents. The best of these would be the burn ointments containing an analgesic. You'll also find numerous burn relievers in the form of creams, liquids and sprays. If the skin is broken, a sterile bandage should be applied to help prevent infection.

Burns are discussed, in the medical profession, as first degree, second degree and third degree. Second- and third-degree burns are *not* the sort of thing that one can handle at home and require the immediate attention of a physician or the emergency room at your local hospital. The milder, first-degree burns can often be taken care of at home.

Typical of this is ordinary sunburn. Obviously, prevention is the best cure, as in the case of any situation that requires first aid treatment. However, the application of any of the burn remedies will bring relief for the sufferer, along with assurance that he'll be more careful in the future. Make certain however, that you treat sunburn with a sunburn remedy, not a tanning lotion as is so often done. The tanning lotion is a preventive that should be applied before spending one's time in the sun.

Among other first aid items you'll want on hand will be the necessary materials for making splints in case a fall results in a broken arm or leg. By splinting and thereby immobilizing you make the affected member you can render the victim a bit more comfortable until professional help arrives. Immobilization also prevents further damage. You can form splints of almost anything available in the house that is sufficiently rigid to serve. A broomstick or mop handle, for example.

And if you live in an area where such things can happen, it would be a good idea to have a snakebite kit on hand. This may appear an unlikely suggestion to those who reside in urban areas, but for those who live in the rural sections of the country, such advice can prove valuable. Wherever in the country you live, insect stings are a constant possibility, and you should check with your physician about this. Some people are extremely allergic to insect stings or bites, and the usual treatment is the immediate injestion of antihistamines. If this is your problem, and your physician so advises, be prepared by having a sufficient supply of antihistamines on hand.

Dog bite is another frequent problem, and while the bite itself can best be treated as any puncture wound, the dangers of hydrophobia remain. It can be avoided, this prolonged and painful series of inoculations, if the offending dog can be captured and brought in for examination. If the dog cannot be located, there is no other course available than to start the treatments at once.

Impact damage (called "trauma") caused by a fall, an accidental blow with a baseball bat, or any of a number of other things can be treated by the application of cold compresses or an ice bag. Failure to administer such treatment as quickly as possible will result in discoloration and swelling. A cold compress will reduce such swelling almost at once and need only consist of a small pile of ice cubes wrapped in a clean towel. Of course, the home that is properly equipped for first aid will have an ice bag that makes such applications a great deal easier and a lot neater.

Learn how to go about administering first aid when a crisis occurs. The American Red Cross offers excellent training in first aid, and we would urge that at least one family member take advantage of this training. The small investment of time could very well save a life. Excellent books on the subject are to be had in almost any library, and again, are well worth the reading.

There are other steps you can take as preliminaries. When was the last time that you and members of your family had tetanus shots? A simple scratch with a rusty nail can cause problems if you aren't protected. These should be renewed about every ten years, because the immunity conferred is long-lasting. More frequent shots are associated with an allergic reaction. Again, by all means, consult with your family physician on this matter and follow his advice.

When a crisis occurs and the problem is one that is beyond your own ken, then call your local physician. If he cannot be reached, contact your local first aid squad or ambulance corps. The local police are usually well trained in this area also.

If all else fails, and you are able to, get to your local hospital's emergency room. That's what it's there for, and chances are that you'll find sympathetic treatment for whatever the problem might be.

Chapter Ten

Wounds

When we talk about wounds, we're talking about anything that punctures or abraids the skin. This can include stab wounds such as administered by a nail; it can include cuts such as you might accidentally receive from a knife or razor blade; it can include scratches, and scrapes, and just about anything that breaks the skin and which may or may not result in almost any type of bleeding.

What you must first do is make an immediate evaluation to determine if medical aid is required. How? Look for dark spurting blood, which can mean that a blood vessel has been severed or punctured, or for any bleeding that cannot easily be stopped. Excessive blood loss is dangerous and requires expert medical attention.

It is important to know how to stop excessive bleeding. Elevation of the wound, direct pressure over the wound with sterile dressings, finger pressure applied to the main artery supplying the bleeding area, a tourniquet applied to the arm or leg are all effective methods of controlling bleeding if the practitioner is knowledgeable, but irreversible damage can be done without proper knowledge, especially in the case of improperly applied tourniquets. The best preparation is a good course in first aid. Short of that, a booklet detailing first aid procedures should be kept with emergency supplies.

Not all wounds will bleed excessively. Small puncture wounds, scrapes and scratches may bleed little or not at all. Some bleeding is beneficial. The blood will help to flush and cleanse the wound. And blood containing the proper amount of hemoglobin will also promote healing.

If you are dealing with a major wound, you will, of course, immediately call for help from your doctor, first aid squad or police headquarters. But small wounds, including cuts, scrapes, scratches and bruises can safely be treated with self-medication, and it is those that we will deal with in this chapter.

How to go about treating minor cuts and bruises is often debated by physicians themselves. The general concensus calls for thorough cleansing of the wound, the application of a suitable antiseptic and then covering the wound with a sterile bandage.

The cleansing of the wound is an extremely critical matter. If any foreign material remains in a cut, gash, puncture or other wound, the chances are that healing will be inhibited until the foreign body is removed. Many such wounds require minor surgical procedures with sterile instruments to effect such a removal. A wound that is suspect should be brought to the doctor's attention, since not to do so may result in festering and infection.

Puncture wounds especially must not be treated lightly, as these wounds often do not bleed freely, and they are difficult to cleanse. Therefore the danger of infection due to harmful bacterial agents (including tetanus) or foreign matter is great. Your physician is best qualified to treat such wounds, and he may decide that a shot of tetanus antitoxin and perhaps penicillin or another antibiotic are in order.

The first step should be the cleansing of the area with soap and water. Following this, flush the entire area with hydrogen peroxide. A suitable antiseptic should then be applied. If the wound appears to continue bleeding, but the bleeding is not profuse, use a sterile gauze pad to cover the wound. Elevating the wound above the rest of the body will help stanch the flow. Now apply a proper covering, using (for larger areas) a sterile gauze pad and then bandage to hold the pad in place.

You'll find many specially treated gauze pads and bandages that will not cling to clotted blood, and these make removal of the bandage easier when it is time to change the dressing. It should also be pointed out here that when a bandage is to be removed, yanking on the adhesive tape can be quite painful to sensitive skins. It's a far better idea to use a bandage to cover both wound and skin, using the adhesive tape to hold the bandage in place, rather than using the tape directly on the skin.

If the skin is badly torn, it may be advisable to use an "H" bandage over the break to reduce the exposed area of the cut. But whatever the condition, it is of utmost importance that a good antibacterial medication be applied to prevent future problems. The wound should be kept covered, and when a scab forms, this should be protected by a cushiony bandage to prevent irritation and secondary infection.

Where children are concerned, near panic can set in if the child sees blood, and this panic can be heightened if you exhibit panic yourself. Try to maintain aplomb (a fancy way of saying "keep your cool") and offer soothing comments while you minister the necessary first aid. Remember that the youngster is hurting, is frightened, and wants reassurance.

If possible, avoid the medications that will sting or burn, for sufficient pain is already there. What is called for is some tender, loving care. At the same time, tend to the hurt.

Many times, we receive what has to be called a "minor cut or scrape." The usual treatment is to react by pulling back, saying "ouch," rubbing the tender area for a moment, and then forgetting all about it. We don't like to baby ourselves by running for the first aid kit to treat a wound so small that by the time you find the antiseptic, you can't even remember where the wound is! In most cases, this is all well and good, and the treatment applied is sufficient to the wound. Small cuts, scratches and abrasions are so commonplace that they're almost a way of life. Surely, we are not recommending that you dash for the antiseptic for each little bump, or you'd probably be spending much of your time worrying these things to death. Small cuts will heal themselves in time, for the body is a very forgiving machine. It takes a great deal of punishment and heals itself.

A small cut can respond beautifully to almost the minimal treatment. Typical is the cut that one receives while shaving with a blade-type razor. Nicks and blade cuts are commonplace, and most men don't even react with pain to these minor cuts. We usually mutter some foul oath and apply a bit of instant first aid in the form of a dab of toilet tissue, which forms an absorptive network over the cut and stanches the flow of blood. We leave home with this mess on our faces, and usually by the time we reach our place of work, the paper is ready to be removed. Those of us who are more concerned about appearances and have the sort of stoic nature to withstand the sting will apply a bit of styptic powder or a styptic pencil. It burns and stings, you dance around in pain, but the blood stops flowing. Stypic, rich in alum, draws tightly, causing the severed capillaries to shrink and stem the bloody tide. You can use styptic on other small cuts and bruises. All you have to do is be able to withstand the momentary pain.

A scrape, incidentally, is much like a burn, and almost instant pain relief can be had by applying cold compresses or soaking in cold water if an extremity is affected. A good antibacterial ointment or salve can be applied, and the scraped or bruised area can be covered.

In recent years, there's been some controversy regarding the treatment of any sort of skin problem with vitamin preparations rather than with purely antiseptic healing agents. A & D ointment, a salve containing both vitamin A and vitamin D, is used extensively by some people to promote healing of minor skin cuts and bruises. Others prefer vitamin E to promote healing, and will purchase capsules of vitamin E which they proceed to puncture with a small pinhole, applying the oil-like substance directly to a cut. However, while these products certainly can't do any harm and might well be beneficial, they should be used only *after* the cut has been properly cleansed and treated with a suitable antiseptic.

Furthermore, we cannot overly stress the need for systemic prophylaxis as well. Even the smallest skin puncture can leave you susceptible to tetanus, and this should not be chanced. See to it that your tetanus shots are up to date, and if they aren't, question your family physician about this.

Another type of bleeding can result from impact, where the skin is not punctured or ruptured, and no external bleeding occurs. Capillaries, those small blood vessels under and through the skin, can be damaged, and the result will be a dark blue mark, called "black-and-blue." This can best be treated by the application of cold compresses or an ice bag. If the injury is to the head, by all means see a physician to ascertain that no damage to the brain has been suffered. If pain persists, a physician should be consulted. There could well be a bone bruise or chip resulting from such an injury.

Nosebleed

Nosebleed is another problem that is fairly common, and while no antiseptics or medications are usually called for, the reason for nosebleed should be investigated. If a nose bleeds for no apparent reason, you should see a physician and find out precisely what the reason is.

One youngster who had frequent nosebleeds accepted them as a matter of course and never really got too excited by the phenomenon. When she had one during the school day, the school nurse and the teachers fluttered about, worrying over the matter. The child simply tilted her head back and waited. "What does your mother do for your nosebleeds?" the nurse asked her. "Oh," the child replied, "she puts tabasco sauce on it." The adults were horrified until she explained that the Tabasco pepper sauce was in a small-diameter bottle kept in the refrigerator, and the icy-cold sealed bottle was held alongside the nose until the bleeding stopped.

Cold is the ideal means to stanch the flow of blood from the nose. The latest and best advice is to tilt the head back, apply a cold compress over the bridge of the nose and another at the nape of the neck. It works almost every time.

Chapter Eleven

Burns and Scalds

Burns are classified by degree of damage and by severity. In *first-degree burns,* the skin is reddened and unbroken, as in simple sunburn. In *second-degree burns,* the top layer of skin is blistered and partly destroyed. Severe sunburn and burning by hot liquids (scalding) are examples. In *third-degree burns,* the entire skin thickness is destroyed or charred, as from burning by flames, with injury extending to tissues beneath the skin. The severity of a burn depends on the extent of body surface affected. *Minor burns* are second-degree burns of less than 15 percent of body area, or third-degree burns of less than two percent of body area. *Moderate burns* are second-degree burns of 15 to 30 percent of body area, or third-degree burns of less than ten percent of body area, except face, hands and feet. *Critical burns* are second-degree burns of more than 30 percent of the body; or third-degree burns of more than ten percent of the body, or of the face, hands or feet, or burns complicated by injury of the respiratory tract, fractures, major soft tissue injury, or electrical burns.

It must be understood that while burns and scalds are labeled almost familiarly as first degree, second degree and third degree, these classifications have some measure of overlap, one with another. If you have sufficient second-degree burns over enough of the skin's surface, it can be as damaging and debilitating as a localized third-degree burn might be.

If the burned area is extensive, or if the burn is second or third degree, if the burn or scald is such that pain is intense, if the skin is broken and bleeding, or if there is no bleeding but the skin is blistered severely, there is nothing in the way of self-medication that is going to help. You must seek a doctor's help at once or pay a rush visit to the hospital's emergency room. Severe burns can result in death.

The remedies discussed in this chapter are for emergency first aid only, to ease the pain until you do get to a doctor, and are meant only for minor or first-degree burns such as sunburn, radio-frequency burns and industrial burns.

The minor burn can be problem enough. There seems to be much confusion regarding treatment, and oddly enough, the age of the person you ask will almost always indicate what the treatment recommended will be! Older people, who can remember the old wives' tales, will recommend that you immediately apply a liberal coat of butter. Younger folks suggest treatment with a tannic acid-based ointment. The latest recommendations are that burns be immediately immersed in icy cold water and kept under water until relief is felt. From what we have been able to gather, this last treatment is the latest and best, for the very covering of the burned area, even though that covering is nothing more than water, will bring instant relief from the pain that comes with a burn.

There are excellent burn remedies available that can be applied directly to the afflicted area, and bandages can be applied over these. However, in the case of burn or scald, keep in mind that the injured skin is very sensitive. A specially treated gauze should be used which will not allow the skin to cling to the bandage, causing even more pain when the bandage is removed to change the dressing or permit a physician to examine the afflicted area.

Sunburn

The best cure for sunburn is prevention, and this can best be accomplished by either avoiding sun or using a suitable ointment or lotion that will screen the harmful sun's rays which can cause severe burning. Be careful in your selection of the lotion, too. While the various oils on the market will keep the skin lubricated and supple, they do not screen out the burning elements, with the result that sunburn can occur anyway. At one time it was thought that a good pigmentation of the skin could be achieved by using a mixture of tincture of iodine and baby oil. However, the iodine merely colored the surface of the skin. No protection was offered at all.

Using a proper screening-type lotion, you should limit your first exposures to the sun to brief periods so that gradual tanning will result. Overdoing things can result in serious sunburn, indeed.

Once you have gotten sunburned, the skin blisters and becomes extremely tender. In time the blisters burst, and when the skin dries out it peels, resulting in a blotchy, discolored appearance that is anything but what you expected when you started out in the first place.

Cooling, antiseptic and analgesic applications are called for at once. Apply a sunburn cream (such as Noxzema) to alleviate the discomfort, with additional applications as required. The soothing emollients will bring fast relief to the tender skin. Other products available in spray cans of various types will eliminate the necessity for even touching the skin. If no such materials are available, relief can be obtained simply by sitting in a tub of cool water, making sure that the affected areas are immersed.

What you are dealing with is a first-degree burn. While sunburn is not normally a serious matter, certain side-effects can make it serious indeed. If sunburn is accompanied by dehydration, nausea, fever or cramps, see a physician at once. The blistered skin should not be picked at, nor should the blisters be burst. Secondary infections can be set up that will lead to more massive problems.

The skin will be sorely itchy, and the temptation to scratch at the skin with the fingernails must be avoided. Instead, apply a good skin cream, and some of the itchiness should be relieved.

In applying any remedies, read the package insert carefully. Be sure the areas around the eyes are avoided in applying these preparations, as some of these products can hurt the eyes if allowed to enter.

Once you have firmly established that common sunburn is all that you are dealing with, it's also a good idea to take two aspirin to help reduce pain.

Radio-Frequency Burns

With more and more people trying to repair their own television receivers and radio transmitting equipment, another type of burn is becoming very much more common — the radio-frequency burn, caused by exposure to high-voltage, high-frequency currents.

What actually happens is rather complex. The electric shock causes muscles to contract involuntarily. The hand that touches the "hot wire" of the TV set will be pulled back as the muscles contract, and may be caught and ripped on a sharp chassis corner or metal part. Severe bleeding can result from this, which will have to be treated in addition to the burn caused when the electricity jumps to the finger.

Electric shock is extremely dangerous, and while the patient may be fully conscious and ambulatory, medical care is of the utmost importance. There are things that can go very wrong with patients who suffer electrical shock, and the burn that appears at the point of contact, while no slight matter in and of itself, can be the very least of the troubles that can occur.

Industrial Burns

Industrial burns, those burns that can occur while on the job, should be treated at once by a physician. Actually, any first aid problems that occur on a job are usually given more and better treatment than burns or accidents of any sort that take place in or near the home. Chances are that this is due to the fact that treatment is more readily available through a company doctor or nurse, or a union steward or foreman concerned for an employee.

Other Burns

In some cases, you're going to have complex burn problems to deal with that are combinations of things. A case in point concerns a young boy who was playing with a wood-burning set. The hot, sharp point of the tool cut his finger, producing a cut wound and a burn at the same time. The burned cut was bleeding, and the boy's father didn't know whether to treat the cut with an antiseptic or the burn with a burn ointment! The offended finger was placed under cold running water which cleaned the wound and relieved the pain of the burn. The next step was a thorough washing with peroxide, and when the bleeding stopped, a bandage, treated first with a good burn ointment, was applied.

Burns can also be caused by caustics or acids. If any of these is accidentally spilled on the skin, the best treatment is to flush immediately with clear, running water and secure the services of a physician at once. Do not attempt to neutralize by using an acid on a caustic, or vice-versa. Burns from these chemicals can be extremely damaging and very, very painful. Continue to flush the area and call a doctor immediately.

Treating Minor Burns

The average burn that you'll have to contend with is the usual so-called "minor burn" that you'll run across in the home. To be sure, there are those exceptions that will occur when a boiling pot is upturned on the stove, or the gas stove decides to ignite suddenly, shooting explosively hot gases back into the room. These things can and do happen, and certainly you should be prepared for them. However, more likely you'll have to contend with burns caused from your electric iron.

The first-degree burn should be treated first by plunging the affected member into cold water. The water serves as a covering and will almost at once help to relieve the pain. Following this, the burned or scalded area should be examined to see if the skin has been broken or blistered. Burn remedies are available in pressure cans so that nothing contacts the skin itself except a mild and gentle relieving spray.

If blistering does occur, do not attempt to burst the blister yourself. Rather, visit your physician for his best advice on the matter. If the blister *has* burst, do not attempt to pull or peel the skin, but rather, again, see your doctor if you can. If not, apply the burn spray and then a spray-type bandage which will help reduce the chances of infection. Keep the area clean and keep an eye on it to see that it heals properly and correctly.

You can help to alleviate the pain by taking a couple of aspirin, but if pain continues, by all means see the physician.

In summary then, burns or scalds of any type are nothing to fool around with, and while the best cure is prevention — exercising a bit of care to keep them from happening — the fact is that they will indeed occur. When they happen, burns should be immediately and properly treated.

There are as many "old wives'" cures for burns as there are old wives, for burns have been around as long as there's been fire and heat. Most of these are about as useless as they can be. As these words are being written, however, we simply know that the next time you come in contact with a burn, somebody is certain to say "put some butter on it."

Don't you do it.

BURN AND SUNBURN

Product (Manufacturer)	Dosage	Anesthetic	Antimicrobial	Other
Americaine (Arnar-Stone)	aerosol ointment	benzocaine 20%	benzethonium chloride, 0.1% (ointment)	polyethylene glycols (ointment) water-dispersible base (aerosol)
Bactine (Miles)	liquid		methylbenzethonium chloride, 0.5% chlorothymol, 0.1%	alcohol, 3.17%; tyloxapol, 0.35%
Butesin Picrate (Abbott)	ointment	butamben picrate, 1%		
Medi-Quick (Lehn & Fink)	aerosol pump spray	lidocaine	benzalkonium chloride	isopropyl alchohol, 12% (aerosol) 79% (pump)
Noxzema Medicated (Noxell)	cream lotion		phenol, over 0.5%	menthol, camphor, clove oil, eucalyptus oil, lime water, water-dispersible base
Noxzema Sunburn Spray (Noxell)	aerosol	benzocaine, 1%	benzalkonium chloride	menthol, 0.1%; alcohol, 7%; emollient
Nupercainal Ointment (Ciba)	ointment	dibucaine, 1%		acetone sodium bisulphate, 0.5%
Solarcaine Foam (Plough)	foam	benzocaine, 0.5%	triclosan	menthol, camphor
Unguentine (Norwich)	aerosol spray	benzocaine	benzalkonium chloride chloroxylenol	phenol, 1%; aluminum hydroxide; zinc carbonate; zinc acetate; zinc oxide; eucalyptus oil; menthol; alcohol 7%
Vaseline First-Aid carbolated Petroleum Jelly (Chesebrough-Pond's)	ointment		chloroxylenol, 0.5%	petroleum jelly; lanolin; phenol, 0.2%
Xylocaine (Astra)	ointment	lidocaine, 2.5%		polyethylene glycols, propylene glycol

Chapter Twelve

Skin Problems

The skin, as a young friend explained, "keeps the insides in and the outsides out." Our concern in this chapter is to deal with some of those things that require medical treatment that we can administer ourselves and to point out the ones that need a physician's care.

The skin, or epidermis, is subject to many problems for which over-the-counter drugs are offered as a palliative. The best treatment for skin problems, of course, is prevention, and frankly, because the skin is always available and well within reach, this is relatively easy to accomplish.

First and foremost, the skin should be kept meticulously clean. Pores, those small openings in the skin, tend to collect oil and dirt and having done so, they can close over this foreign matter, sealing it inside where it can cause festering and infection in the form of pimples and other eruptions. The skin should be carefully cleansed every night with a hot, soapy water which is thoroughly rinsed away, then a good-quality astringent bath should be used, followed by a thorough rinsing with cold water to close the cleansed pores.

This is especially true where the skin is oily. However, if a dry skin is subjected to this sort of treatment, it can dry out to the point of becoming scaly.

Soap and water, of course, will be your strongest ally in the fight against skin problems, but there are some problems that require additional preparations, and we will discuss those in this chapter.

Acne

There is a dichotomy in our society, for while youth is king, and we all like to present to the world a youthful, blemish-free complexion, one of the major skin problems known, *acne vulgaris,* is peculiar to the young. There are numerous forms of acne, and these should, in each case, be brought to the attention of a physician for his recommendations.

There are several types of preparations for acne, and in one form or another, all are beneficial. While no real cure has yet been found, the problem seems to be one of generating surplus skin oils and the blackheads that result. The oils attract and hold dirt. If the blackheads are removed, the skin overgrows the swollen pore, infection occurs and the ugly pustules form. There is a vacuum device available that will remove the blackheads safely, but prevention of formation is the far better method. If the pustules are permitted to dry in the subcutaneous zone and are then squeezed through the skin, an enlarged tear in the skin occurs where the pustule was removed, and this remains as a permanent facial scar.

The best and safest method is thorough cleansing. The application of a good ointment with a zinc oxide base to assist in drying the skin thoroughly will help.

In selecting an acne medicine, keep in mind that you are purchasing a medication and not a cosmetic. While some of these medications contain cosmetic coloring to blend with the skin — and that's all right — remember to check the list of active ingredients to be sure that there is more to the product than a mere cover-up.

Introduction to Chart

If you are not troubled with acne, this chart will not have great meaning to you. However, if you *do* have acne you'll find it most helpful.

You plan to purchase an acne medication. Look at the ingredients for each product and see if there are any that you know yourself to be allergic to. Eliminate those products as possibilities.

Now decide on the form that you prefer, a gel, cream or liquid. Of the one you like best, compare the ingredients, and then select the one with the ingredients that you want that is offered at the lowest cost.

If you own druggist does not have the medication that you want, have him order it for you. If he tries to tell you that another product is "the same," simply show him the differences on the chart!

ACNE PREPARATIONS

Product (Manufacturer)	Form	Sulfur	Resorcinol/ salicylic acid	Antibacterial	Other
Aconomel (Smith, Kline, French)	cream cleanser	8% 4%	resorcinol, 2% (cream) 1% (cleanser)		
Benoxyl (Stiefel)	lotion				benzoyl peroxide, 5%-10%

Betadine Skin Cleanser (Purdue-Frederick)	cleanser		povidone-iodine 7.5%	
Clearasil Medicated Cleanser (Vick)	cleanser	salicylic acid 0.25%		alcohol, 43% allantoin, 0.1%
Contrablem (Texas Pharmacal)	gel	5%	resorcinol, 2%	alcohol, 9.5%
Cuticura (Purex)	ointment	precipitated	8-hydroxyquinoline	petrolatum, mineral oil, mineral wax, isopropyl palmitate synthetic beeswax, phenol, pine oil, rose geranium oil
Epi-Clear (Squibb)	lotion	10%		alcohol, 10%
Listerex Herbal Lotion (Warner-Lambert)	cleanser	salicylic acid 2%		polyethylene granules surface-active cleansers
Medicated Face Conditioner (MFC) (Mennen)	liquid	salicylic acid 1%		alcohol, 55%
Microsyn (Syntex)	lotion		resorcinol 2% salicylic acid 2%	sodium thiosulfate 8%, colloidal alumina, menthol, camphor
Multiscrub (Bristol-Myers)	cream	2%	salicylic acid 1.5%	soapless detergents, polyethylene resin granules, 26%
PhisoAc (Winthrop)	cream	colloidal, 6%	resorcinol 1.5%	alcohol, 10%
PhisoDerm (Winthrop)	cleanser			entsufon sodium, petrolatum, lanolin, cholesterols
Thera-Blem (Noxell)	cream	2%	resorcinol 1.5%	phenol 0.5%	menthol, 0.5% camphor, 0.5%

Psoriasis

Psoriasis is a severe hardening and encrustation of skin patches, which scale away, leaving angry red spots. Unchecked, these ugly spots can even become infected and can run. The sight of psoriasis is unpleasant, the patchy areas become extremely itchy, and the temptation to scratch at them and pick away the hard, scaly skin is very real. Unfortunately, this can lead to secondary infection, and the transfer to other areas of the skin. Psoriasis will appear at the scalp, the knees and the elbows, although in severe cases, no part of the body is immune.

Sadly, as of this writing, the cause is unknown, and no cure as such exists for psoriasis. Among the many self-medicating drug products you will find numerous salves and ointments that will provide a measure of relief from the itching and scaling. But this medication must be continued as long as the affliction lasts. Should you be thus afflicted, by all means consult your physician. He will recommend the proper course of treatment and will, at least, offer some relief from the effects and symptoms. Be wary of those who claim a "sure cure," for there is none.

Your physician will recommend one of the balms that will relieve the itching and flaking, but do not attempt to remove the scales with the fingernails, tearing at the areas where the scales are affixed to healthy skin. This will result in bleeding and possible infection. To help relieve the itch, use a good moisturizing agent and keep the area clean, washing with tincture of green soap. After rinsing, pat dry (do not rub) with a soft towel and then apply the regular medication. Another excellent aid is to wash the area with Phisohex or Phisoderm liquid soap. Phisohex was formerly sold over the counter, but the Federal Government now requires that it be sold by prescription. Phisoderm can be obtained without a prescription.

Occasionally a quack cure for psoriasis appears, but until the product or process is approved by the FDA, do not experiment or allow yourself to be experimented on. We indulged in such an experiment recently.

Having a mild case of psoriasis at the elbows, we were induced to make a comparison test, using a medicated cream on one elbow and a moisturizing agent alone on the other. In less than two weeks the elbow treated with the moisturizing agent was almost fully healed, exhibiting no sign of patchiness. The one treated as regularly with the medicated cream exhibited no improvement whatever and was indeed, sore to the touch.

It has also come to our attention that scientists at Harvard have developed excellent treatments for psoriasis and this, too, should be investigated.

Warts

Warts are a virus infection and take many forms. The usual treatment is to burn them away, which is done by a physician at his office. A local anaesthetic is injected, or a chemical freezing agent is sprayed on, and the wart is removed by a high frequency electronic device. This is the best state-of-the-art methodology available today.

Some people insist on treating warts themselves, and some of the things they attempt are actually frightening. Some people, untrained, and unable to recognize warts as such, simply think that they are encrusted skin, and pick at them until they bleed. Others treat them by abrasion, using lava stones meant for callous reduction.

Because any unusual skin growth might be a harbinger of cancer, you would be best advised to make your first stop your local physician for his opinion. Chances are that if he agrees that your problem is no more than a wart, he might even recommend a patent remedy as a curative. Do give him the opportunity to do so, however.

Many of the problems that occur with the skin will require a physician's attention and in most cases, self-medication is futile. Some of these problems are readily curable by proper medication. They can also be symptomatic of more serious problems and are therefore sufficiently serious in and of themselves to warrant medical attention.

If you attempt self-medication, you'll come upon a product called Preparation W which is as good as anything for the problem as we've come across. The product will after repeated direct applications to the wart eventually eliminate it. The usual chemical product used is a mild formalin solution, and you'll generally find formalin in any wart preparation you might buy.

In General

Such skin problems as shingles, which is a virus infection, and eczema can and should be corrected by a physician, since any attempt at self-medication can, at best, provide only temporary relief.

Callouses are hardened growths of skin that usually occur where there is friction or wear. It is the body's way of protecting skin surfaces that are subject to such erosion. Callouses can occur on the heels or on the edges of the toes or on the hands where tools are used excessively. Skin-softening medications are the best way to reduce these, and foot soaks with an iodine base are another. However, you can purchase abrasives such as lava and pumice stones that will erode callouses down to the proper layer of epidermis. What you ought *not* to do, is cut, slice, or clip this "dead" skin, for you have no way to know how deeply to go and might well remove live skin also, which can induce bleeding and possible infection. If the problem is sufficiently severe, by all means consult an orthopedist, who can correct the condition properly.

Another important skin problem is athelete's foot. This is a highly contagious, very uncomfortable condition and should be corrected as soon as it is recognized. Begin by a thorough washing and careful drying, and then the application of any one of the remedies for athelete's foot. We have found such products as Desenex or Absorbine to be the sort of thing that will help, short of a prescription product. Whatever else you do, avoid direct contact with things that other family members might come into contact with. Towels used for drying the victim's feet should be washed in hot, hot water before being used by others.

The important thing about athelete's foot is that it should be cured and not simply neglected. Like so many other problems that man is heir to, it won't simply "go away" without treatment. It will spread and become more intense.

Fever sores, the result of coryza or the common cold, are treated with a number of combined analgestic/antiseptic medications. Those used for the treatment of other inflamed mucosa will do nicely. One that is eminently effective is a type which has a drying agent in it that promotes healing by eliminating runniness.

Typical of skin problems that may afflict is the matter of bad foot odor. This can strike anyone. You can wash and scrub the feet until they are raw, bathe the feet several times a day, and still be so afraid to remove your shoes in public that you're reluctant to go to a shoe store to buy a new pair of shoes. It's certainly not humorous to the person so afflicted.

There are many preparations available to mask foot odor, and there are shoe inserts to absorb foot odor. While these may or may not work to your ultimate satisfaction, they are well worth trying. A friend who was so afflicted finally took the problem to a podiatrist, who explained that there were several possible treatments, but that these must be tried in succession to find the one that would work. The treatment began with a yellowish liquid in a small plastic bottle. One capful diluted in hot water was to be used as a foot soak twice daily. When the bottle was finished, so was the problem. Our delighted friend asked what the substance was, and the podiatrist explained that it was formic acid. "We simply burned away the sweat glands on your feet!"

Sound like a drastic solution? Perhaps it is, but the problem was drastic too, and a drastic solution was called for. Our friend now kicks his shoes off at every opportunity, just to relax.

While not essentially a skin problem, hemorrhoids are classed as such by many people who do not understand them, so we are including them here. Hemmorhoids are basically varicose veins. The problem is excruciatingly painful and an embarassing one to speak about, for they occur at the anus. Elimination becomes difficult or painful, the hemorrhoids can bleed, and even walking can become a source of irritation. They itch severely, and even when the feces are soft, elimination can still be painful.

Until recently, the approved procedure was surgical. By cutting the hemorrhoids away, a cure was effected. In recent years, however, a totally new procedure was devised in which the offending hemorrhoids are simply tied off and allowed to dry and fall away. The procedure is less painful and recovery is a good deal faster.

Short of this sort of treatment, the best advice we've gotten is to apply an analgesic balm or a suppository containing pain relievers. These, such as Preparation H or Ointment Americain, will reduce the pain, diminish the itching and promote healing.

Skin dryness or over oiliness, while not necessarily a medical problem, can be uncomfortable and can lead to other problems if not properly cared for. If you do nothing to relieve dryness, flaking can occur. Oiliness, if not properly taken care of, can result in clogging of pores, followed by the collecting of foreign matter in the pores, and then acne.

The usual solution is to treat the symptom rather than the cause, and while this may provide temporary relief, the problem will have to be constantly treated or the symptoms will continue to recur.

The right way to handle this is to seek the help of a physician, who can usually correct matters by adjusting diet or providing supplemental vitamins or additives that will effect a cure.

However, until you get to the doctor, you might as well have some relief for the problem, and dryness can be corrected by the addition of any of the available moisturizing creams that will — if the skin is dry — be absorbed like ink into a blotter. The correct way to use these is to continue the application until the skin simply refuses to absorb any additional. At this point, the excess can be blotted up, and the itching will stop, skin comfort will again be realized.

Excessive oiliness requires the application of any of the astringents which will dissolve and remove the excess oils. The astringent should be applied with a cotton ball, allowed to sit on the skin surface for a moment or two, and then should be washed away with soap and water used in ample quantity.

These problems are usually caused by an imbalanced diet, and again your physician can usually prescribe the right chemicals to correct the imbalance and then gradually reduce the drugs and permanently correct the situation with a proper diet. You should not simply dismiss the problem by saying "Oh, I have oily skin."

There is another problem that man is heir to, and that is dandruff. While it may appear, symptomatically, to be dry skin, it is actually a flaking and a hardening of patches of skin surface. However, what you might simply analyze as dandruff could be the beginning of seborrhea or psoriasis. Once the fact has been established that it is indeed dandruff, it can probably best be treated with one of the commonly available dandruff shampoos.

There are many available preparations to treat dandruff, to stop the flaking and itching that accompanies it. The products used are generally sulphur-based astringents and the products generally available for this will do a fine job of eliminating the problem.

Every once in a while, you may notice a small, angry pimple on the skin that seems to have appeared for no apparent reason whatever. A bit of pressure relieves the problem, and chances are that you will soon forget all about it. Usually the problem is an ingrown hair, a hair whose follicle or root, for some reason, is upside-down in the skin's surface. The hair, buried inside the skin, causes a small local infection to appear, and when the hair is removed the problem ceases to exist. You can recognize this, for the protruding hair is usually not as long as the hairs adjacent to it. If you are able, remove this hair with tweezers before serious festering can begin.

Men, in particular, are subject to a similar, somewhat serious problem called the pilonidal cyst. This is a pimple filled with blood and sera (clear body fluids) as well as pus, and it occurs at the base of the spine. Sometimes this can be relieved by the application of a bit of finger pressure, but the only true and permanent removal is by surgery. The surgery involves about a week's hospital stay, but this is far better than the alternative, which is agonizing pain and no real relief.

In colder weather, you will find some specific skin problems. First and foremost is the matter of chapped lips, caused by coldness, dryness and wind. To protect your lips from chapping, your best bet will be to keep the lips and mouth covered. Ski masks may not be the prettiest things in the world, but they do the job nicely. You can also protect the lips by the liberal application of a good lip balm. Interestingly enough, in the case of chapped lips, the remedy is the same as the preventive. You simply apply the lip balm, which moisturizes the dried skin on the lips and restores suppleness and lip comfort once again.

As the skin dries when the lips become chapped, there is a temptation to peel away the dead skin. This should not be done. The skin on the lips is soft and tender, and the dead skin is liable to take along live skin with it. The result can be severe bleeding and secondary infection.

Ingrown toenails, not usually recognized as a skin condition, can be dreadfully painful and can even prevent proper walking. This condition should be tended to by a professional. A podiatrist will usually taper the nail down to the quick, and then the properly tapered nail can grow out straight, pushing the skin aside as it emerges. There is a limit as to how far you can trim your own toenail, and you should not attempt this.

Should you have only a mildly ingrown toenail and want to attempt self-medication, there is a product called Outgrow. It is applied by a glass dropper, and it will toughen and harden the skin, causing the nail to emerge straighter. The product also contains analgesics that will deaden the pain at the sensitive area. Self-medication is in order, provided that sharp points of nail matter are first removed and then the tender underskin is hardned by chemicals. Again, this product cannot correct a severe case of ingrown nail, which can only be done by a physician or podiatrist. If in doubt, by all means visit your physician.

Chapter Thirteen

The Mouth and Teeth

Fortunately, you'll find ample over-the-counter medications to correct many problems that exist in the mouth, not the least of which are problems occuring with the teeth.

However, we must again issue the warning that many of the problems are simply symptoms of more serious underlying problems, and merely to mask them with the patent remedies available is not going to quiet the major problem that may be present. The matter of sore and painful teeth, for example, can be corrected by the judicious application of a topical or systemic analgesic. Unfortunately, by doing this instead of visiting your dentist, the ultimate outcome might be an extraction instead of just a filling. The sudden occurrence of bad breath can ordinarily be controlled by proper use of a suitable mouthwash. But that same bad breath might be the harbinger of a more serious gastrointestinal problem, with the breath odor nothing more than symptomatic of the more serious problem.

The remedies suggested in this chapter therefore are for the solution of acute and not chronic problems. The chronic problems require the aid of a good physician or dentist if they are to be properly treated and cured.

Toothache

Naturally, the first mouth problem we think of is toothache, and if there is pain, its source must be identified. Should the pain be localized, by all means make plans to see your dentist. However, until you can make the visit, there are certain things you can do to alleviate the pain.

First, take one of the systemic analgesics such as aspirin, Tylenol or Datril. There is a common misconception that the analgesic should be applied directly to the sore area, and as mentioned we have known people to chew and swallow the aspirin, washing the dissolved product over the tooth area for better effect. The fact of the matter is that for these products to work at all, they must first be swallowed and taken into the bloodstream. Topical application, rinsing powdered aspirin over the sore area, will do absolutely no good whatever. One packager produces an aspirin in chewing gum form, and while that is all well and good, it is only after the aspirin has been swallowed that it can be of any help.

We all suffer on occasion from teeth that have become sensitive to pressure, chewing, hot or cold. The feeling is most uncomfortable, and while the usual analgesics will help, a good corrective for this is a product called Sens-O-Dyne toothpaste. One young lady we know suffered from highly sensitive teeth, to the point where she wanted her dentist to extract all of them and relieve her pain. We learned that her dentist suggested the Sens-O-Dyne toothpaste, that it be applied liberally over all the tooth surfaces and then wait for half an hour before brushing the teeth. She now uses this product regularly, and is "cured."

When a specific tooth is giving pain, perhaps because of an untreated cavity, temporary relief can be had by the topical application of a liquid remedy called Anbesol. This comes in a small bottle with an applicator rod in the cap. Relief is felt almost at once, but unfortunately this relief is short-lived. Treatment will have to be repeated again and again until the tooth is brought to the attention of a dentist.

Another topical analgesic comes in the form of a poultice that is immersed in warm water and then applied directly to the offending tooth. It is placed between the tooth and gums and held in place to continue to provide relief for a longer period of time.

Many of the problems that occur in the mouth are caused by the very nature of the mouth and its function. Foods are introduced, during the chewing process saliva is added, and the food, after chewing, is passed to the stomach for further digestion.

In chewing, foods are ground and impacted, and particles lodge in between the tooth surfaces. Some of these food particles are difficult to dislodge, but unless they are removed they will begin to disintegrate where they are, swelling and becoming more firmly lodged in place, and as they decompose, they will give off an offensive odor and can start the formation of caries (cavities).

These food particles must be removed by proper cleansing. After meals, a thorough brushing with a stiff toothbrush and a good dentifrice should be administered. Dental floss should be used, and if one is available, a mouth-irrigating device should be employed. There is no reason why a toothbrush and dentifrice cannot be carried to the office for use after lunch. Finally, rinse thoroughly with an antibacterial mouthwash.

Dentures

People who wear dentures will find, in time, that the skin surface under the denture will recede, causing the possibility of the denture shifting. While this can be compensated for by having the dentist reline the plate, until this is done, the shifting may abrade the tender skin, causing irritation. At the beginning, this can be corrected by using one of the new plasticized denture adhesives, but when sufficient time has elapsed, relining becomes essential.

If you are unable to get to your dentist, you can buy a temporary lining material at your local drugstore. This is immersed in hot water, pressed into position on the inside surface of the plate, and then trimmed. The plate is put into position in the mouth, you bite down hard for a few minutes and then trim the excess material once again. When you do get to your dentist, he can peel this material away and do a proper job of relining the plate.

Proper cleansing of the dental prosthetic is important. It should be removed from the mouth twice daily, soaked in a good commercial denture bath and then scrubbed thoroughly with a denture cleanser and a denture-cleaning brush. Most dentists today do not want their patients who wear dentures to keep them out all night, soaking the denture in a glass of water. This can result in the remaining natural teeth shifting during the night and creating major problems. The denture wearer should simply remove the plate(s) twice a day while performing other ablutions, and then replace them both for the day and for the night.

In any event, do not overlook a regular, daily treatment with a suitable antibacterial mouthwash. This, of course, applies to everybody, regardless of whether or not dentures are worn. It is especially necessary to people who have partial, permanently mounted bridgework, for food particles can easily lodge between the gum surface and the prosthetic.

The regular use of mouthwash will do more than just freshen the breath. It rinses away lodged food particles, sweetens the breath and leaves you secure in not having to guard your breath when in close contiguity with others.

If you find that the average mouthwash is too intensely flavored for your own taste, dilute it with a bit of water to ease the sharpness of the taste, but then rinse more often to see that a sufficiency of the product is used.

If you are able, don't hesitate to gargle with the product as well, to cleanse the mouth all the way back to the throat.

People who are often in close contact with others can carry a small vial or bottle-type dispenser with a breath deodorant in liquid form that can be used almost any place and whenever the need arises.

There are certain things that must be avoided. People who are subject to rapid growths and collections of tartar (also called calculus) will observe that when they go for their semiannual dental visits and cleanings, the dentist removes this buildup by "scaling" the teeth. He uses a sharp tool and actually flakes this material away, picking and scraping at and below the gum line. They may attempt to supplement his regular treatments by doing this themselves at home, using a pin or needle. All it takes is a single slipup, and you're in for a mouthful of trouble.

Incidentally, there's one old wives' tale that really does work as far as oral pain is concerned. If you'll check the labels of some of the liquid pain relievers, you'll see that they are basically tinctures, or mixtures rich in alcohol. It is the alcohol that provides the relief from pain. It used to be (and still is) recommended that a mouthful of some spirit be held in the mouth over the affected area. In time, when relief was felt, the spirit could be swallowed and the process repeated when the pain returned.

This does work. The alcohol has a numbing effect on the tooth where it touches topically, and inside you where the effect is systemic! Maybe it won't actually cure the problem, but after a few applications, the problem won't seem quite as pressing in any case.

Oral problems must not be left to chance. When you see a problem beginning to develop, visit your dentist. Calculus, for example, can quickly and easily be taken care of by the dentist as a part of the regular semiannual cleaning. If it is not taken care of, the gums will recede from the irritation, and this will result in a gingivitis problem that is not reversible. Once the gums begin to recede, there is no way to bring them back again.

Many of the chronic mouth, teeth and gum problems can be attributed to assorted vitamin deficiencies. Only your physician and dentist can correct these problems for you, providing the necessary identification of these deficiencies and administering corrective doses of these vitamins to correct such problems and keep them from recurring. In addition, cancer of the mouth and gums can be easily detected by your dentist, and if you visit him regularly, such conditions can be pinpointed and corrected early on.

The message is obvious.

Visit your dentist regularly, and keep your mouth in good, clean and healthy condition.

Introduction to Chart

What kind of mouthwash do *you* use? Most people have one that they favor, but usually for the wrong reasons. Most people select a mouthwash on the basis of taste, then secondly for effectiveness.

If you will look up your own mouthwash on this chart, then compare the ingredients with those of another, you may find that you are able to buy an equally effective mouthwash at a lower price. You might also learn that the mouthwash you are using is by far not the best for you.

MOUTHWASH Ingredients

Product (Manufacturer)	
Astring-O-Sol (Breon)	tincture of myrrh, methyl salicylate, alcohol 70%, zinc chloride
Chloraseptic (Eaton)	Phenol, sodium phenolate
Colgate 100 (Colgate-Palmolive)	benzethonium chloride 0.075%, alcohol 15%
Lavoris (Vick)	zinc chloride 0.22%, alcohol 5%, cinnamaldehyde and clove oil 0.06%
Listerine (Warner-Lambert)	menthol, boric acid, thymol, eucalyptol, methyl salicylate, benzoic acid, alcohol 25%
Scope (Proctor & Gamble)	cetylpyridinium chloride, domiphen bromide 0.005%, alcohol 18.5%, glycerine, saccharin, polysorbate 80, flavor
S. T. 37 (Calgon)	hexylresorcinol 0.1%, glycerin

Chapter Fourteen

"Eye, Ear, Nose and Throat"

Certain physicians specialize in what is called "EENT" which stands for "Eye, Ear, Nose, Throat" and the trend is toward even further specialization. In some cases, the problems that these areas are heir to can be self-medicated. However, a word of warning is in order, for these openings to the inside of the body require careful treatment.

The most important thing to remember about treatment is that if your attempt at self-medication does not bring instant relief, see a physician at once.

The Eye

The human eye is a wondrous mechanism that provides you with sight and with depth perception, and you need both of your eyes to get along properly in this world. When the eye becomes tired, this will be manifested by redness. You can treat the redness and tiredness with special eyedrops available for that purpose. Use these according to the dosage instructions on the label and certainly no more frequently than recommended. Because the eye surface wants to be moist at all times, the inner eyelid usually provides the liquid lubrication required. The eyedrops serve to supplement this, usually bringing rapid relief from dryness.

When more concentrated treatment is called for, a liquid eyewash and an eyecup are recommended. The eyecup is filled to the proper level, placed over the eye with the head tilted down, and then the head and eyecup are brought smartly upward so that the liquid can wash over the entire eye surface. The eyelids should be held open as widely as possible and the eye moved about inside the eyecup, so that all surfaces of the orb are exposed to the liquid.

Did you know that people's eyeballs, regardless of their size of body or weight, are essentially the same size? Because of this, eye bath cups are all of a size, and you needn't worry about this aspect in making a purchase. However, the eye bath cup used to be available only in glass, but can now be had in an assortment of plastic materials that makes them less expensive and more convenient. In purchasing an eye bath, be certain that the edges that press against the facial skin are smooth and free of molding kerfs — those little rough edges. At least one packager of eye bath solutions provides an eye bath cup with a cap molded on the opposite end. When you get the product at home, you remove the bottle cap and screw the eye bath cup to the top of the bottle. This keeps the bottle closed, and the eye bath convenient for when it is needed.

Any excessive discharge from the eye might be the product of a serious eye infection and should be brought to the attention of a physician at once.

When you are fitted for eyeglasses, the optometrist might suggest a test for glaucoma. The usual fee for this additional test is very low and can well help to save your sight. By all means have this test made, especially if you are over 35 years of age. Should you find that your eyes tire easily and often, yet you have not been doing a great deal of close work, by all means visit your ophthalomologist. If you see your family physician about such a problem, chances are that he will recommend such a visit himself.

Glaucoma, or an increase in intraocular pressure, can be caused by eye problems directly, or, it might be the result of heightened blood pressure. Either condition is worth knowing about, and the test for glaucoma can reveal the condition.

Since many people wear contact lenses these days, you'll find an assortment of plastic containers to store the lenses, marked "L" for left and "R" for right. You will also require a suitable cleansing bath for your lenses, and your own ophthalmologist or optometrist will recommend the best for your own use. Because the composition of the lenses will vary, and as the lenses are easily damaged and susceptible to scratching or abrasion, we suggest that you consult with your doctor first, even though the cleaning liquids are available over the counter.

The Ears

The human ear is another problem area for people. One of our advisors states that "the only thing you should ever put in your ear is your own elbow!" However, while this does state his case, there are some ear problems which require that you take steps and measures to correct. One of these problems is the buildup of ear wax. If this is not removed, the buildup can ultimately block the opening to the inner ear and cause deafness. There are numerous means that people employ to remove ear wax, from paper clips and hairpins to ear spoons and rubber syringes to flush the wax away! Such activity can result in serious damage to the hearing mechanism and should be avoided. The safest way to remove earwax is to use a liquid eardrop that is allowed to settle in the ear and then is removed along with softened, loosened wax with the aid of a cotton-covered swab. Even this must be used with great care, for the inner ear is easily approached through the ear opening, and can easily be permanently damaged.

Within the inner ear are small, string-like hairs that operate to bring sound into the ear and to the brain. Excessive irritation can dislodge these hair-like nerve endings. They are frequently sensitive, and the finest conduct the higher frequencies to within. You may find that high frequencies are those that you lose first. Many modern youngsters who subjected themselves to loud, raucous rock and roll music have sacrificed their ability to hear these higher frequency sounds. People who live in large urban areas and are subjected to loud impact noises on their jobs have also suffered such hearing loss.

Most physicians recommend the use of ear stopples to prevent such damage, and the scientists who work in the area of noise pollution research use these all the time. The best type is a rubbery plastic that fits snugly inside the ear, with a sound-sensitive flapper valve that will close to protect the ear from impact noise. When such noise approaches the ear, the valve closes to protect the ear by reducing the amount of such noise that is permitted to enter. No hearing loss at normal levels is caused by such devices.

Water can enter one's ear while swimming, and this will result in some discomfort when the swimmer emerges from the water. You've surely seen people at the side of the pool, hopping up and down on one leg with heads tilted askew. This ridiculous dance could be avoided with the use of proper ear stopples designed to keep water out of the ear.

The hairs that are in and around the ear are there for a purpose. They keep foreign matter from entering the ear by filtering it. Granted that very little in the way of foreign matter is available these days, for the encroachment of nature has been all but been eliminated in our present urban civilization. However, we have replaced those few undesirable elements that nature thrust upon us with more, equally undesirable man-made matter such as soot and dust. To further complicate matters, society dictates that hair in and around the ears is not to be tolerated. As a result, we shave, clip and otherwise attempt to remove this natural protective shield. While we have no argument with society on this matter, we do object to the means used by some people to attain this end. Sharp scissors can inflict untold damage and should not be used. Care should be exercised at all times.

Where a hearing loss does occur and is irreversible, the obvious solution is a hearing aid. Such units are relatively inexpensive and can be made so that they are all but invisible. Small, flesh-colored plastic devices concealed behind the ear with a clear plastic tubing to a molded earpierce inside the ear can function ideally to help restore hearing. Where there is damage to the ear itself and the audio nerves are still functioning, bone conduction hearing aids can still do the job.

Most of the firms that sell and install hearing aids maintain shops where the units are on display, and they usually have facilities to administer audiometer tests that will show you just how serious your hearing loss is, and where in the frequency range it occurs.

The portion of the hearing aid that goes inside the ear must be molded specifically to your ear in clear plastic. A properly made and fitted unit is as much your own as a prescription drug is meant for you. Do not simply assume that you can borrow somebody else's hearing aid to try out, any more than you can borrow eyeglasses or false teeth!

Once you have been fitted properly with a hearing aid, it's going to require periodic maintenance in the form of battery replacement. How should you go about buying batteries for a hearing aid? There are some simple rules.

First and foremost, do not stock up on a year's supply! The batteries have what is called a "limited shelf life" and can decay, just sitting around waiting to be used. Similarly, they can decay just as rapidly on the dealer's shelf. We prefer to buy in shops where they have a large turnover, thereby insuring that you are getting fresh stock.

This does not mean that you ought not to have a few spares around just in case, and you should learn how to change your own batteries, as a matter of course. You'll have to buy the batteries that fit your unit. Size and polarity are important, so be sure to install them right-side-up. You'll find full instructions in the manual that came when you bought the aid. You'll also find a small, limited choice available to you within your size and voltage range. The new alkaline-type cells cost a bit more per battery, but they do not deteriorate on the shelf and actually retain almost full performance until they are put into service — and then last almost ten times as long! The manufacturer's name is not of much consequence, but stick with the better-known brands for more reliability. Our own experience has been that the cheaper imports are a good deal less expensive, but as standards are not as well maintained, they do not hold up as well.

The Nose

This brings us to the nose. The selfsame criticisms levied against the ear must also be directed toward the nose. Scissors used to remove nose hairs, the corner of a razor blade, all are to be shunned. The actual pulling or plucking of nose hairs should also be avoided. It's not only painful, but can result in infection.

One of the things that can cause you to try self-medication for the nose is stuffiness that can impede proper breathing. This can be caused by any number of things, ranging from the simple common cold to serious allergy problems. A severely stopped-up nose can cause you to breathe through the mouth, causing the oral mucous membranes to dry out, and the result is a sore throat over and above the nose problems. For self-medication, you will find a wide variety of over-the-counter medications that will provide relief in a great number of cases.

One way to obtain relief from a stopped-up nose is to take an oral decongestant in the form of capsules, pills, tablets or liquids. It is of the utmost importance to remember that many of these remedies contain antihistamines that induce sleepiness. Be extremely careful while taking these that you do not attempt to operate machinery or drive a car.

Since oral decongestants require a little time before they take effect, in the interim or in place of the decongestants you may wish to use nose drops or sprays directly on the clogged membranes, softening mucous so it can easily be expelled and reducing the swelling to help clear the passages. By clearing the normal flow passages, postnasal drip can be reduced, and the throat will benefit from this.

Unfortunately, for every good there's always a warning! Please read the dosage instructions on the label carefully. Too much of these nasal drops or sprays can cause overdrying, and serious problems can result if you exceed the dosage directions.

Some medications are in the form of creams or unguents to be applied directly to the nostrils, and others require the use of a vaporizer. This gadget generates steam, which is mixed with chemicals and then is inhaled to provide relief. Naturally, such a device cannot be easily carried about and used publicly, but there are small pocket inhalers which can help when you are away from home.

Problems with the eyes, ears, nose and throat can be indicative of problems that are systemic and are really located elsewhere in the body. This is a two-way street, too. Problems in breathing might *not* be nose problems, but simply a manifestation of serious pulmonary infection. Possibly even worse. And rest assured that discomfort in the eyes, ears or throat might be but manifestation of more deep-seated troubles that no amount of self-medication can allay.

The point is that when discomfort or pain is present, and this discomfort or pain does not respond to self-medication, you *must* see a physician and permit him to treat the problem at its source, a source that you may not even be aware of. Sure, maybe your troubles are manifested by a tenderness or soreness or even a sharp, acute pain. It's entirely possible that treating the problem where it appears to exist will eliminate the problem. Our only point is that if you use self-medication and it doesn't help, by all means seek out competent professional assistance so the problem can be eliminated.

The Throat

The throat, coated with mucous membrane, is susceptible to a number of ills that are treatable by self-medication. The type of self-medication that you use will be dictated by the problem itself. If you find a hoarseness, a slight "tickle" or a mild sore throat, chances are that the problem will respond to any of a number of mildly analgesic throat lozenges that are taken by allowing them to dissolve on the tongue. Where more concentrated application of the medication is required, you will find numerous liquid medications that, although they act in the same fashion, are usually more effective and longer lasting. The effective ingredient in such remedies is one or another of the analgesics which act by numbing the surface.

Where these cannot be used, gargles are frequently found to be effective.

Throat lozenges usually contain analgesics, along with natural products such as oil of wintergreen, oil of eucalyptus, mint, and/or menthol. These are in a gum arabic base, or something similar, and act as emollients for the sore and reddened tissues.

Aspirin can also be used for sore throat, for it is a pain depressant. However, do not attempt to dissolve the tablet and gargle with it, spitting out the used solution. Aspirin is a systemic analgesic, not a topical one. The only way for such treatment to do any good at all is to swallow the liquid after gargling.

In treating a sore throat by yourself, be extremely careful. This is especially true where children are concerned. Without a proper diagnosis by a physician, there is no way to be certain that you do not have an infection such as tonsilitis, or even worse. Infected tonsils can be treated by antibiotics these days, or, on the decision of your physician, they can be surgically removed. Should you elect to minister to the child yourself, you may find that the simple sore throat should have had proper medical care, and having been allowed to linger untreated, worse damage can occur. Don't take unnecessary chances.

Generally speaking, throat problems as well as any other medical problems are symptoms. Your physician will check these symptoms in combination with other symptoms that you may have, and on the basis of such checks, can usually arrive at a conclusion and a diagnosis. For example, sore throat by itself, with any other symptoms being absent, might simply be the result of strain or overwork of the throat and its environs. Sore throat plus fever could indicate an infection of some sort that requires not just an analgesic, but an antibiotic that cannot be obtained without a prescription. Now let's assume that you elect to treat the sore throat with aspirin. Aspirin also masks body temperature (and is indeed a specific for the reduction of body temperature). If you decide ultimately to visit your physician, inform him that you have been taking aspirin, so that he might not overlook the possibility of infection when he finds no fever present.

Certain other specifics that are not medicines (such as Grandma's remedy — a spoonful of honey) may not be as much of a healer as some of the drugstore products, but they provide relief for a while, anyway.

Because sore throat is usually coupled with other problems such as cough or cold, you'll find numbers of remedies that treat the sore throat as well as the other symptoms. Our recommendation is to first determine what the basic problem is, and then treat that. If you've been shouting, singing, or talking a great deal and have a sore throat as a result, there is no need to treat anything *but* the sore throat.

Coughing can cause a soreness in the throat, for the tussive action of the cough is indeed irritating. To take a local analgesic without eliminating the cough is futile. Any of the cough remedies or antitussives will supress the cough and probably contain a mild analgesic as well.

Frequently coughing can be caused by a collection of phlegm at the back of the throat, or by postnasal drip. Both can be relieved by the use of the proper medications. Antitussive medications are either decongestants, which dry the area, or expectorants, which produce additional moisture, enabling you to bring up the offending phlegm. While one is suitable for eliminating the cough, the other might serve only to irritate or compound the problem. Be certain when you purchase a cough medicine that you're getting the one that will do the best and fastest job for you.

There are two types of cough, too. It will help you to recognize which is bothering you, so that you can select the right sort of medication.

The dry, hacking cough, such as heavy smokers suffer, is completely nonproductive. The productive cough is one that removes the phlegm from the throat and windpipe, bringing up clogging sputum and producing a measure of relief.

Expectorants can be of great help where coughing is the result of a collection of phlegm. The expectorant loosens and reduces the phlegm, permitting you to eliminate it by expectoration.

If you have a suitable antitussive cough syrup in the house, bought fairly recently for another family member, there is no reason why it could not be used by a second family member evidencing the same symptoms. However, prescription medicines are meant *only* for whom they were first prescribed.

One of the most common maladies that we all suffer at one time or another, and one for which modern science has not as yet found a "cure," is the common cold. What is the best that we can hope for? To find a remedy that will sufficiently mask the symptoms of the cold so that we forget that we have it until it is healed.

You'll be faced at any drug counter with an assortment of medications that purport to be combinations of ingredients, all-night remedies, eight-hour remedies and pain relievers with agents to dry the sinuses, shrink swelling membranes and allow you to ("ahh!") breathe again! These remedies are all excellent for what they do. The type that you, personally, will swear by is the one that does the best job for you. However, a process of elimination is required to make that determination. In any case, be certain to restrict yourself to the proper dosages according to the label, and *do not take more than one of these at a time.* It's absolute nonsense to take a remedy containing a full dose of aspirin, and then take another with the same thing. If you do, you'll be overdosing on the aspirin.

Another word you should know is "spansule." This is a timed-release medication that works slowly, releasing its active ingredients over a time period specified on the label. It's important that you understand and adhere to the dosage requirements.

Our best information to date is that a cold must run its course. There's an old saying that if you treat a cold and take care of it with proper care and medication, it will only last two weeks. If you try to ignore it, it won't go away for 14 days.

Maybe medical science has not as yet pinpointed the cause of colds. Maybe we still don't know how to treat them. But we certainly have a sufficiency of medications to choose from that will so completely mask the symptoms you'll really forget you have a cold.

Annabel Hecht

This lady, a staff writer for the FDA's Office of Public Affairs, put together a fantastic document that talks about the common cold. So thorough-going did we find this that we include it here in its entirety.

The Common Cold: Relief But No Cure

Had you lived in ancient Rome you hight have sipped a broth made by soaking *Allium cepa* — an onion — in warm water to relieve the symptoms of the common cold. In Colonial America you might have relied on pennyroyal tea or an herbal concoction made from such unmedicinal sounding plants as sage, hyssop, yarrow, black cohosh, buckthorn, coltsfoot, goldenseal, cubeb berries, or bloodroot. In grandma's time, lemon and honey was a favorite recipe, or in extreme cases, a hot toddy laced with rum — the amount of same determined by the age of the drinker.

Today, if you don't have an old reliable remedy to fall back on, you might take one of the literally thousands of drug preparations available without prescription. Some contain ingredients reminiscent of the folk medicine of the past; others are formulated with sophisticated chemical creations. Old or new, simple or sophisticated, many of these remedies will relieve some of the familiar cold symptoms, such as stopped up nose or hacking cough. But not a single one of these products — on which Americans spend an estimated $700 million a year — will prevent, cure, or even shorten the course of the common cold.

So says a panel of non-Government experts called on by the Food and Drug Administration to study the safety, the effectiveness, and the accuracy of claims made on the labels of some 50,000 cold, cough, allergy, bronchodilator, and antiasthmatic drug products. The Panel is one of 17 set up by FDA to examine all nonprescription (over-the-counter) drugs marketed in the United States. The project, mandated by a 1962 Amendment to the Food, Drug, and Cosmetic Act which requires that all drugs be proven effective as well as safe, will eventually lead to the establishment of definitive Federal standards on ingredients and labeling claims for all nonprescription drugs.

The Panel indicated that proper use of nonprescription drugs can be effective in relieving cough, sinus congestion, runny nose, and some of the other symptoms associated wth colds, allergies, or asthma. But it made clear that although these products may relieve certain symptoms they will not cure any of these conditions.

One aspect of this class of drugs that concerned the Panel was the relative scarcity of single ingredient products on the market. This is particularly true of cough and cold remedies. The common cold is a self-limiting respiratory infection which lasts from one to two weeks. It usually starts with a sore throat, sneezing, and runny nose. After a few days, the nose becomes stopped up and the eyes become watery. This is followed by lethargy, aches and pains, and sometimes a slight fever. Cough may occur in the later stages. Often these symptoms do not occur at the same time. Nevertheless, almost 90 percent of cough and cold products now available contain a combination of ingredients intended to relieve a number of different symptoms. Only 46 of the cough-cold products examined by the Panel consisted of a single active ingredient.

The Panel said it is "irrational" to take a combination product unless each of the ingredients is necessary to relieve the patient's particular symptoms. Moreover, because of variations in individual reactions to drugs, fixed combinations may not be suitable for some people. Consumers need more choice in selecting the appropriate treatment for their symptoms, the Panel said, and recommended that all products to relieve cough and cold symptoms be available in both combination and single ingredient form.

Another area of concern to the Panel was labeling of cough and cold remedies. It said labeling for these products "tends to be overly complicated, vague, unsupported by scientific evidence, and in some cases is misleading." The Panel called for an end to claims that one product is superior to, stronger than, or contains more active ingredients than another, or is specially formulated. Under its recommendations such words as "cold medicine," "cold formula," or "for the relief of colds" would be banned from drug labels. Such claims suggest the product will cure a cold when the best it can do is relieve specific symptoms, the Panel said.

One of the most distressing symptoms of the common cold is sore throat and many nonprescription drug products claim to provide relief for this condition. The Panel noted, however, that sore throat can be due to serious infection which should not be treated by self-medication. It recommended that labels on cough, cold, and related nonprescription drugs limit their claimed effectiveness to "minor throat irritation" and should advise consumers to seek medical help for serious throat problems.

Timed-release formulations also came under the scrutiny of the Panel, which found advantages and disadvantages in this type of medication. Obviously it is easier to take one pill instead of two or three, especially at night, but variations in the rate at which ingredients dissolve, differences in individual patient reactions, and even technical flaws in the manufacturing process could mean that the medicine could be absorbed erratically or possibly all at one time. Therefore, the Panel recommended that a four-year period be allowed for industry, in cooperation with FDA, to develop suitable tests for the standardization of all nonprescription timed-release cough-cold products and that timed-release claims not be permitted in labeling unless such claims have been documented.

Children represent a substantial portion of the consumers of cough and cold remedies, yet the Panel found that information on how these drugs affect them is "negligible or non-existent." Lacking definitive data, the Panel sought the advice of a group of experts on pediatric drug therapy in developing the following recommendations: the dose for children 6 through 11 should be half the adult dose, and for youngsters 2 through 5 it should be one quarter of the adult dose. Asthma and cough preparations should not be taken by children 2 through 5 in any amount except on the advice of a physician. Any product with an alcoholic content of more than 10 percent is not for children under 6, the Panel noted.

As for infants up to 2 years of age, the Panel said dosage should be determined by a physician and the labels on nonprescription drug products should make this clear. Labels should never carry a recommended dose for these youngsters unless the product has been demonstrated to be safe for them, the Panel said.

In reviewing all cough, cold, allergy, bronchodilator, and antiasthmatic nonprescription drug products, the Panel studied some 90 active ingredients. These ingredients were divided into six groups (plus a miscellaneous classification):

- Antitussives, which are cough suppressants.

- Expectorants, which help bring up mucus in the bronchial airways so that it can be spit out.

- Bronchodilators, which enlarge the bronchial passages to make it easier for people with asthma to breathe.

- Anticholinergics, which dry up watery secretions in the nose and eyes.

- Nasal decongestants, which open up the nasal passages.

- Antihistamines, a class of drugs used to relieve sneezing and watery and itchy eyes, usually associated with hay fever and other allergies.

Each ingredient reviewed was placed in one of three categories:

Category I — Generally recognized as safe and effective and not mislabeled.

Category II — Not generally recognized as safe and effective or mislabeled. Such ingredients and labeling claims will be removed from products within six months after FDA issues its final regulations on cough, cold, and related nonprescription drug products.

Category III — Available data insufficient to permit final classification at this time. The Panel recommended that when FDA issues its final regulations ingredients which are placed in this category be permitted to remain on the market for a stipulated length of time if the manufacturer immediately begins tests to satisfy the questions raised by the Panel.

Lucky is the cold victim who has only an annoying tickle in his throat or a stuffed up nose. The Panel found 7 ingredients both safe and effective as cough suppressants and 14 safe and effective as nasal decongestants. It recommended that one of the cough suppressants and four of the nasal decongestants which are now available only in dosage levels that require a prescription be made available in effective dosages that could be sold without a prescription.

Not so fortunate is the person whose cough is "nonproductive" or produces only small amounts of thick phlegm. Not one ingredient was found by the Panel to be both safe and effective as an expectorant. Similarly, the Panel found no ingredient both safe and effective as an anticholinergic to relieve watery secretions of nose and eyes.

Fifteen of the ingredients it studied are not generally recognized as safe and effective for cough and cold symptoms and should be taken off the market, the Panel reported. One of these is chloroform, which FDA already has banned on the basis of evidence that high doses of it can cause cancer in test animals.

A wide array of ingredients — 52 all told — were considered by the Panel to be safe enough, but further proof of their effectiveness in relieving coughs and stuffy or runny noses is needed. Scattered throughout the list are names reminiscent of patent medicines and home remedies of the past: cod liver oil, slippery elm, cedar leaf oil, horehound, camphor, menthol, and oil from the koala bear's favorite food, eucalyptus leaves. The Panel recommended that these familiar remedies — as well as the rest of the 52 whose effectiveness it questioned — be permitted to stay on the market for from three to five years if their manufacturers undertake further tests to prove (or disprove) that grandma knew all along what was good for the sniffles.

As for the labeling of cough and cold remedies, the Panel recommended that cough suppressants be permitted to claim that they temporarily relieve coughs due to minor throat irritation, help to quiet the cough reflex, or help you to cough less. But the labels should warn that a cough may be a sign of a serious condition and that a physician should be consulted if it lasts more than one week. The Panel also recommended a warning that cough suppressants should not be used for persistent or chronic coughs such as occur with smoking, asthma, and emphysema. In such cases, coughing is essential to rid the bronchial airways of mucus and other secretions. Cough suppressant labels should not refer to lung or chest conditions, the Panel said, nor should they claim the product works by soothing the bronchial passages.

The Panel said expectorant labels should be permitted to claim that the product helps loosen phlegm or rid passageways of bothersome mucus, but it called for a warning against taking expectorants for persistent chronic cough associated with smoking, asthma, or emphysema, or if there are excessive secretions, except under the advice of a physician.

Labels on anticholinergics could promise temporary relief of watery nasal discharge, or runny nose or watering of the eyes, but such statements as "clears nasal passages" or "opens airways" would not be permitted under the Panel's recommendations. Consumers should be warned not to take anticholinergics if they have asthma, glaucoma, or difficulty in urinating, the Panel said.

Topical nasal decongestants, those applied directly in the nose, present a unique problem. These drugs help clear up stuffy noses by constricting enlarged blood vessels in the nasal passage. But if they are used for too long a time or too frequently they can have the opposite effect and actually enlarge, rather than constrict, the blood vessels. Therefore, the Panel recommended that labeling for topical nasal decongestants warn users not to exceed the recommended dosage and not to use the product for more than three days. If symptoms persist, a physician should be consulted.

Oral nasal decongestant labels should warn against use by persons suffering from high blood pressure, heart disease, diabetes, or thyroid disease unless under a physician's supervision, the Panel said. And products that are inhaled should carry the caution statement: "Not for use by mouth."

Approximately six million people in this country suffer from asthma, a disease marked by wheezing, coughing, and shortness of breath. Many of these people use nonprescription drugs called bronchodilators to help them breathe more easily, and the Panel found 12 ingredients safe and effective for this purpose. Five of them are now available only by prescription, and the Panel proposed that they be changed to over-the-counter status.

Because of variations in the way the body breaks down the two types of drugs most often used as bronchodilators, the Panel said that single ingredient preparations are more effective and safer to use than combination products. It also cautioned that bronchodilators not be used unless a diagnosis of asthma has been made and then only under the supervision of a physician.

Because bronchodilators can have adverse effects on the circulatory and central nervous systems, they should carry labels warning against use by persons suffering from high blood pressure, heart disease, thyroid disease, diabetes, or enlargement of the prostate gland, the Panel said. Labeling also should warn the patient to seek help immediately if symptoms are not relieved in one hour — or in 20 minutes in the case of epinephrine taken by an inhaler. Bronchodilator labels should be permitted to claim that the product is for temporary relief or symptomatic control of bronchial asthma only, the Panel recommended, and there should be no suggestion that it will relieve hay fever or have any effect on the nasal passages.

The relief of hay fever should be left to the antihistamines, the Panel indicated. It found 11 ingredients from this class of drugs safe and effective for relieving the symptoms of allergic rhinitis, or hay fever. Four of these are now available by prescription only, but the Panel recommended that that be approved for over-the-counter sale. Two antihistamines now used in hay fever products require further testing to demonstrate their effectiveness, the Panel said.

Although the antihistamines that are rated safe and effective have a low potential for side effects and toxicity they may cause drowsiness, the Panel pointed out, and it said this fact should be made known on the label. The label also should include a warning against use by people who have asthma, glaucoma, or enlargement of the prostate gland unless under the supervision of a physician.

Acceptable label claims for antihistamines should be that they are for the temporary relief of runny nose, sneezing, itching of the nose or throat, and itchy and watery eyes as may occur in hay fever, but not for the relief of nasal symptoms, such as stopped up nose, nasal stuffiness, or clogged up nose, the Panel said.

Although antihistamines are widely used in the treatment of common cold symptoms, the panel said there is "little valid evidence" that they are effective for this purpose. Claims that antihistamines are effective for cold symptoms have not been substantiated by appropriate research, the Panel said, but it suggested ways these drugs could be tested for the common cold.

The Panel considered a number of ingredients which are often found in nonprescription cough-cold preparations, but which did not fall within the six main categories under review. These included antihistamines added to some cough-cold products as a sedative or sleep-aid. The Panel questioned the validity of adding an antihistamine to a cough or cold preparation for purposes of sedation and recommended that such combinations be taken off the market. But it said combinations that include an antihistamine "for restful sleep" should be allowed to stay on the market provided testing is undertaken by the manufacturer to establish an effective dose.

The Panel also called for additional testing to prove the effectiveness of caffeine, which is added to some cough-cold products to counteract drowsiness caused by other ingredients, and phenobarbital, which is added to offset central nervous system stimulants.

Label claims that vitamins, when used either alone or in combination with other products, are effective as cold preventives or cures should not be permitted, the Panel said. But the Panel added that manufacturers should be allowed to use vitamin C in cold products for three years if they want to do so in an effort to demonstrate its effectiveness, on the condition that no claims are made about the vitamin C.

The Panel's report, the culmination of three years of study of this vast array of ingredients, is advisory in nature. It was published by FDA in the *Federal Register* to allow for comments from industry and consumers. After reviewing the report and the comments on it, FDA will issue final standards for acceptable ingredients and labeling claims for cough, cold, and related over-the-counter drug products. As a result, many products may have to be reformulated and labeling and advertising claims may have to be changed, a process which may take place even before the final standards are issued.

Chapter Fifteen

Mucous Membranes

Mucous membranes fall into a gray area, for they are not hidden inside the body, nor are they exposed, skinlike, to the elements. They do, however, serve as a junction between those internal body elements that are hidden and the tougher skin which is exposed. You'll find mucous membranes at all of the body openings. It is a moist surface that must be kept moist. The problems that can occur in mucous membranes are such that special treatment may be required when difficulties arise. Because the mucous membranes are the way they are, it's almost like dealing with internal bodily organs.

The delicate tissues of mucous membranes can easily be irritated and become inflamed, resulting in severe discomfort and possible infection. Any problem with the mucosa should be brought to a doctor's attention. Should you have a problem in this area and a physician is not available, there are certain things that you can do to provide temporary relief.

If you have a cold, for example, the mucous membranes can swell and inflame, resulting in difficulty in breathing. The nasal passages feel clogged, you have to breathe through your mouth to get any air at all, and as a result of that, the throat membranes will become dry and irritated.

The best way to cure this is first to get your doctor's recommendation and then to take one of the decongestant remedies that will reduce the swelling of the membrane-covered tissues. Check, too, to see if you shouldn't also be taking an antihistamine.

Decongestants act to dry the mucosa. You will find that it's a good idea to take one of the cough drop troches, as this will help keep the mouth and throat lubricated by inducing the additional flow of saliva.

Should the throat become clogged, you may want to try an expectorant which will induce increased liquid flow and thereby help to clear the throat. However, since decongestants and expectorants work to opposite effect, these should not be taken at the same time.

The mucous membrane at the nose, especially at the nostrils, can become infected for any of a number of reasons. The constant expulsion of excess mucous can irritate this area, as will the pulling of nostril hairs. There are a wide variety of nose drops that can act to soften encrustations, making them easier to remove. However, these should only be used in accordance with label instructions and should be discontinued in the event that any adverse symptoms seem to occur.

In extreme cases, the vaporizer will be found to be beneficial, and this should be brought into play if required.

Children must also be watched carefully when in the throes of a cold, for a child can panic when unable to breathe. It's a frightening thing for a youngster, and he should be calmly told to open his mouth and breathe that way, the adults in the vicinity showing no signs of alarm to further frighten the child.

The Mouth

Mouth tissues are also covered with mucosa, and we have all experienced the problem of inflammation in this area at one time or another. We have had our salivary gland orifices inflame, we accidently bite down on a bit of cheek tissue, or we burn our mouths with a particularly hot bit of food.

The tongue can withstand a good deal more heat than the fingers can, and while lay people seem to be unaware of this, magicians take advantage of it. They insert alcohol-soaked balls of flaming cotton into their mouths, they spew live flames across a room and even extinguish glowing cigarettes on their tongues!

Rest assured that if you burned your tongue on a bit of super-hot food, chances are that you could not have held that morsel in your fingers!

The best curative for burns of the mouth, provided that they are minor burns, is to hold a mouthful of cold water over the burned area. Considering the several burn remedies available, there are none that are suitable for use in the mouth! You will note that the cold water almost immediately relieves the pain, and frankly there is little more that you can do for such a burn or scald. An analgesic throat spray might also be used for relief. If the burn is severe, by all means, consult a physician and do not attempt self-medication.

Vaginal Itching

While we do not claim any direct experience with this, we have been informed that it can drive a person up the nearest wall, resulting in an immediate visit to the doctor. This appears to be one problem that does not get put off. Neither should it be put off. It can be a symptom of more serious problems and, if chronic, should be brought to the doctor's attention.

If, on the other hand, it occurs only periodically or occasionally, there is no reason to put up with the discomfort. The immediate relief that can be obtained by scratching can result in secondary infection, compounding the problem. The best corrective for temporary itching is the application of a palliative such as Ointment Americain. When the itching has passed, you may want to try one of the douches which will have a fine, salutory effect. Should the itching recur, see your physician at once.

The Rectum

Rectal itching is another problem that can be caused by any of a number of things, most of which will require the attention of a physician before a permanent cure can be had.

A typical example would be worms. This can be diagnosed by submission of a stool sample, and it can be cleared with proper systemic medication. However, all rectal itching is *not* a sign that you have worms! It can be caused by the ingestion of highly spiced foods, or by simple irritation.

This sort of problem can usually be alleviated by the application of an analgesic balm. If the situation persists or recurs, see your physician. Should the problem be one of diet, this can usually be corrected by changing the diet, or avoiding acid or highly spiced foods.

Sometimes the problem results from the failure of the bodily organs to properly neutralize such foods. In other cases, bodily imbalances can cause excretions that can prove irritating. The restoration of proper balance should be accomplished by corrective chemical treatment under your doctor's supervision.

One thing that has proven eminently effective in such cases is the use of activated charcoal in capsule form. The charcoal is adsorptive of such bodily poisons, renders them harmless, and ejects them, along with the charcoal as part of the eliminative process.

Where analgesics are used, these can be applied in the form of creams or gels, or internally in the form of analgesic suppositories. In either case, by all means read package directions, and understand that the normal eliminative bodily processes will remove the analgesic too. The application of such analgesics *after* elimination will extend the value.

The Eyes

Mucous membranes also appear at the corners of the eyes. This is an extremely tender area, and one that is exposed to all sorts of dust, grit and the goo that fills the air, especially in our urban areas. When irritated or tired, the eyes should be carefully flushed with a suitable eyewash, or if no eye bath is available, with proper eyedrops.

For the most part, mucous-covered tissues of the body are delicate and extremely tender, deserving of the greatest respect. If you plan to use self-medicating drugs, consult your physician first. Do not attempt to duplicate any applications by taking one item internally and another externally at the same time unless label directions recommend this.

A lot of mucous membrane problems will occur during other bodily upsets. If you have a severe head cold, you may find that your nose, throat and eyes are where everything seems to settle. One manufacturer of pharmaceuticals advertises is "Don't trade your headache for an upset stomach!" You may find that some of the cough tablets, taken orally, will bring blessed relief to your throat, only to play havoc with your stomach and intestines when they reach those organs.

Apply a bit of common sense. Know what you can take and what you can't. Do not fly into panic and bow to discomfort by reaching for anything that promises relief, regardless of consequences.

While mucous membranes appear at all openings to the interior of the body, you do not treat all mucous membranes in precisely the same way. The treatment is determined by which mucous membrane you have to worry about, and if there is any shred of doubt, by all means see a physician.

HEMORRHOID PRODUCTS

Product (Manufacturer)	Dosage	Anesthetic	Antiseptic	Emollient Lubricant	Other
Americaine (Arnar-Stone)	suppository ointment	benzocaine 280 mg (suppository), 20% (ointment)	benzethonium chloride, 0.1%	polythylene glycol base	
Lanacane (Combe)	cream	benzocaine	phenylmercuric acetate 0.02% chlorothymol	water washable base	resorcinol
Nupercainal Ointment (Ciba)	ointment	dibucaine, 1%			acetone sodium bisulfite 0.05%
Preparation H (Whitehall)	ointment, suppository		phenylmercuric nitrate 0.01%	shark liver oil, 3%	live yeast cell derivitive supplying 2000 units of skin respiratory factor
Vaseline Hemorr-Aid (Chesebrough-Pond's)	ointment			white petrolatum, 100%	

Chapter Sixteen

Your Lungs and Breathing

Quite frankly, most lung and breathing problems require that you speak to your physician. However, once he has made a diagnosis, chances are that he will recommend one of the over-the-counter breathing aids to treat asthma or related conditions, where breathing is impaired by swollen membranes. The medications we're talking about are not inhalers, but they expel a jet of medicine that is taken directly into the lungs to relieve such problems as asthma.

They are held to the lips, the cap is pressed, and a deep breath is taken through the mouth. Used regularly (but only under a doctor's advice to correct a specific fault) they will reduce inflammation, permitting easier breathing.

For milder problems, you can buy an inhaler over the counter. This is a small plastic device, tapered at the top, containing papers that are treated with medications. You insert the plastic cap into a nostril, hold the mouth and other nostril closed and take a deep breath. The air is drawn through the inhaler into the nostril, where decongestants can do their work on nasal passages and sinuses. Do not use these to excess. They must be used no more frequently than every three or four hours.

The breath enters the lungs through the nose and mouth, through the trachea and into the lungs. Blockages of any of these passages can cause breathing problems. Sometimes these blockages can be caused by swelling or growths on the surfaces of the various canals, other times by the accidental inhalation of foreign objects. In most cases, self-medication can be undertaken, but a physician must be consulted first, just in case.

Be extremely cautious about children and their breathing problems. You'll be absolutely amazed at how ignorant children can be of such matters, and more than one youngster has shoved a bean or pea into a nostril only to forget about it. If there are any problems with children's breathing apparatus, by all means see a physician and get things straightened out under his care.

Noxious vapors can be totally invisible and can be inhaled even without your own knowledge. Should you feel ill or queasy at any time, consider the possibility that you may have inhaled some gas. Again, a physician should be consulted at once.

Illuminating gas, that used for operating gas ranges, is always mixed with a strong odor to help identify it, for such gas has no odor of its own. If you detect this odor in your home, by all means telephone the local gas company which will immediately dispatch a repair crew to locate the source of the leak and rectify it.

Remember that you have but one set of lungs, and you have to take excellent care of them if you expect them to last your lifetime. If you observe any serious problem, such as difficulty in respiration, a hacking cough, or deep-seated sputum or blood in the sputum, consult your physician at once. Many problems, even the most serious, can be corrected with proper medication.

If you work in an area where there is excessive dust or chemical dust, by all means wear a respirator mask that will filter the dust out of the air you are breathing.

Snoring

One of the most common breathing problems is one that occurs at night, in the form of snoring. Usually the person who snores is not at all disturbed by his own nocturnal soundings. It's those obligated to sleep with the snorer that will suffer.

Snoring is caused by the soft, fleshy cap which covers the glottis, serving to stop up the air passages when eating, so that food will not be inhaled into them. As you breathe in your sleep at night while you are supine, this flap can vibrate, creating the typical snoring sound. When you are awake, an involuntary control takes over, keeping this flap from moving, and you do not snore. There have been attempts to remove this flap surgically and thereby eleminate the problem. In fact this is done on certain animals. But in humans the procedure is not recommended, as it will introduce an element of danger.

In some cases, all that is required is a shift of positions to stop the snoring, and this is certainly worth experimenting with. One manufacturer produced a hard rubber ball that is meant to be pinned at the back of the snorer's pyjamas. If he rolls over on his back, the ball should waken him, he should shift his position to his stomach or side, and the snoring should stop. As we said, this works in some cases, but not in all.

Smoking

Smoking is a habit with little or nothing to recommend it. Yet stopping is next to impossible once the habit has seized you, for the withdrawal symptoms are very real.

The craving for nicotine seems to settle in the kidneys. One very real aid to stopping is called Bantron, a small, white pill containing lobeline sulphate. You take this pill according to package instructions, and it helps displace the nicotine collected in the kidneys, flushes it away, replaces it with a non-habit-forming product, and eliminates the desire for cigarettes. The package instructions will also tell you to take regular and frequent showers to wash away the nicotine that is expelled through the skin surface and pores.

At the same time, start carrying your cigarettes in another pocket so that you can't simply reach for them as you used to. Wanting to smoke will require a genuine effort to reach into a unfamiliar place. Throw away your cigarette lighter and do not carry any matches so that you must actually ask for a light when you want to smoke. Make smoking as inconvenient for yourself as you can. Explain to friends and family that you are trying to quit. They will commiserate and avoid smoking in your presence as much as possible, making it easier for you. Go to places where you will be unable to smoke. If you go to a movie, sit in the nonsmoking section.

The lobeline sulphate has an astounding effect on your smoking habits. If you attempt to quit completely, this will help you tremendously. If you just want to cut down, the desire to smoke will be almost eliminated, and when you do reach for a cigarette, chances are that you'll take one or two puffs and then put the cigarette out.

The stuff really works and, if you want to stop, will make the stopping as easy and as comfortable as it could be.

Vaporizers

The vaporizer is an excellent aid where congestion impedes breathing. This is a mechanical device that provides excellent relief, if properly used. It is very much like a pressure-operated tea kettle, in that liquids are placed in the proper chamber, the chamber is sealed, and the unit is plugged into an electrical outlet. A heater inside the unit heats the liquids to the point where they boil and turn into steam; this steam is loaded with the required medications and can be inhaled directly. The units are usually completely safe as long as the directions in the instruction book that comes with the unit are followed.

When purchasing such a unit, make sure that it is a type approved by Underwriters' Laboratories. You can tell this by looking for the little green stick-on label that identifies it as such an approved product.

COLD AND ALLERGY

Product (Manufacturer)	Dosage	Sympathomimetic	Antihistamine	Analgesic	Other
Alka-Seltzer Plus (Miles)	effervescent tablet	phenylpropanolamine hydrochloride 26.5 mg	chlorpheniramine maleate, 2.1 mg	aspirin, 324 mg	
Allerest (Pharmacraft)	time capsule	phenylpropanolamine hydrochloride 50 mg	pyrilamine maleate, 15 mg; methapyrilene fumarate, 10 mg		
Bayer Decongestant Tablet (Glenbrook)	tablet	phenylpropanolamine hydrochloride 18.75 mg	chlorpheniramine maleate, 2 mg	aspirin, 325 mg	
Contac (Menley & James)	time capsule	phenylpropanolamine hydrochloride 50 mg	chlorpheniramine maleate, 4 mg		belladonna alkaloids, 0.2 mg
Coricidin-D (Schering)	tablet	phenylpropanolamine hydrochloride 12.5 mg	chlorpheniramine maleate, 2 mg	aspirin, 325 mg	
Coryban-D (Pfipharmics)	capsule	phenylpropanolamine hydrochloride 25 mg	chlorpheniramine maleate, 2 mg		caffeine, 30 mg

Product	Form				
Dristan (Whitehall)	time capsule	phenylephrine hydrochloride 20 mg	chlorpheniramine maleate, 4 mg		
Neo-Synephrine Compound (Winthrop)	tablet	phenylephrine hydrochloride 5 mg	thenyldiamine hydrochloride 7.5 mg	acetaminophen 150 mg	caffeine, 15 mg
Sinarest (Pharmacraft)	tablet	phenylephrine hydrochloride 5 mg	chlorpheniramine maleate, 1 mg	acetaminophen 300 mg	caffeine, 30 mg
Sine-Off (Menley & James)	tablet	phenylpropanolamine hydrochloride 18.75 mg	chlorpheniramine maleate, 2 mg	aspirin, 325 mg	
Sinutab (Warner-Chilicott)	tablet	phenylpropanolamine hydrochloride 25 mg	phenyltoloxamine dihydrogen citrate, 22 mg	acetaminophen 325 mg	
SuperAnahist (Warner-Lambert)	tablet	phenylpropanolamine hydrochloride 25 mg	phenyltoloxamine citrate, 6.25 mg thonzylamine hydrochloride 6.25 mg	acetaminophen 325 mg aspirin 227 mg phenacetin 97.2 mg	caffeine
4-Way Cold Tablets (Bristol-Myers)	tablet	phenylephrine hydrochloride 5 mg		aspirin, 324 mg	magnesium hydroxide 125 mg, white phenolphthalein, 15 mg

Chapter Seventeen

Your Digestive System

In this chapter we're going to discuss some problems that affect your stomach and digestive system. Included in these are hyperacidity, diarrhea, constipation and gas, and we'll talk about these in relationship to the over-the-counter medications that can help them.

Hyperacidity

The most common complaint where the stomach is concerned is hyperacidity. This goes under many other names, all of which will be nontechnical and familiar to the layman. It's called variously "heartburn," "indigestion," or "gas," or — if you are of Italian extraction — *"agita."*

How important is this? Over $42.5 millions were spent in 1971 on advertising for antacids. According to Product Management Magazine, the total volume of sales for antacids in that same year was $108.8 millions. Certainly more than sufficient gas to take care of our national energy crisis!

What should be considered, as far as this particular malady is concerned, is that many of the symptoms readily mimic the symptoms of far more serious illnesses, and sometimes it's hard to tell the difference. The same gastric pain that is causd by hyperacidity can be caused by such serious problems as acute gastritis, pancreatitis, angina, gallstones, hiatus hernia, or pulmonary or cardiac infarction.

The point is that by chewing and swallowing that little antacid tablet, you may not be curing a condition that you have self-diagnosed as "heartburn." Your best remedy in some of these cases would be to seek competent medical help at once.

A leading pharmacist who teaches at the Rutgers College of Pharmacy made the point very clearly. He eats carefully, and as a result rarely if ever has heartburn. If he should suffer the stomach and chest pains that would indicate this problem to those of us who are less discriminating in our selection of foods, he would immediately consult a physician. He suggests, on the other hand, that the person who constantly suffers the discomfort of acid indigestion would be better advised to take an antacid and then, should the discomfort not to be relieved, visit a physician.

As you will learn, there are several common forms of active ingredients available in antacid tablets and other similar remedies. The various manufacturers offer these products, each with a different active ingredient, which are usually available under various trade names and in different dosages.

Usually the product, no matter what active ingredient is used, cannot perform until it reaches your stomach. Therefore the factor of solubility comes into play in making a choice.

Of course, the best cure of all is the avoidance of those foods and condiments which will produce gas and which will induce hyperacidity. Barring that, you must decide which forms of the antacids are most convenient for you. If you prefer the tablets or powders that are to be dissolved in water, consider whether or not water will always be available. If you prefer the chewable tablets, experiment with these to find the ingredient that will work best for you, and then select from those available containing that ingredient to find the one that is most pleasantly flavored and that will chew most readily. Time the relief so you can decide on what works best for you.

Another problem with antacids is that some of them can have a harmful effect on some people. Should you find any negative side effects as a result of taking a particular antacid, discontinue the use of that product and try another. Should you continue to meet with bad results, by all means consult your physician.

It must again be stressed that many of the symptoms of heartburn are the same as symptoms of more serious illnesses, and whenever a shred of doubt exists, by all means see a physican. If you're having a heart attack, no amount of antacid is going to correct the situation.

Constipation

Another common stomach malady is politely referred to as "distress in the lower tract." Constipation can leave you uncomfortable. What's more, when constipation is finally relieved, the first elimination can actually be painful. As an almost-solid wall of feces moves through the S-shaped bend in the lower intestine, the unyielding, unrelenting mass causes this bend to distend out of shape, resulting in pain. And then as this almost-solid wall of feces is forced through the anal opening, the resulting tissue stretching can cause a great deal of pain.

There are several forms of laxatives available. The most common type simply acts to increase the rate of peristalsis — the pulsation that causes feces to move through the lower intestine. Other types act on the feces themselves, to loosen and lubricate, to facilitate elimination. Some laxatives actually do both.

As with most self-prescribed medications, you must find out which will work best — and most comfortably — for you.

The basic soap-and-water enema might be the most efficient, and at the same time the most inconvenient. Suppositories are also efficient, and, although somewhat less convenient, are certainly easier to use than enemas.

The most common laxatives available today are to be had in chocolated form, in pill form, as chewing gum tablets and even in the form of liquids. The ideal of course, is to find one that works best for you. What does "best" mean? You want a laxative that will operate at a time most convenient for you, and not catch you short at the last minute in a desperation situation. You want a laxative that will operate without causing undue pain over and above.the pain and inconvenience of constipation; and you want a laxative that will be relatively easy to take and be pleasant tasting. In the old days, it was fashionable, when a cathartic was required, to dose people with castor oil or mineral oil. With the wide variety of pleasant tasting, scientifically operating laxatives known to man today, this sort of thing is utter foolishness!

Diarrhea

The direct opposite of constipation is, of course, diarrhea. This is usually accompanied by severe cramps and an almost incontinent liquid bowel movement. The lower intestine is usually severely irritated, and if left unchecked, a general feeling of weakness can result. If simple drugstore remedies do not correct the condition, a physician should be consulted at once.

The best cure, of course, is to correct the cause. If certain foods or fruits are the cause of this condition, then cut down on the intake of those comestibles. Frequently, a change of water can cause this problem. Travelers to countries south of our own borders call this "Montezuma's Revenge."

Where chemicals must be injected to correct diarrhea, you'll find an assortment of tablets and liquid emulsions that calm the problem quickly and leave a "coating" on the wall of the stomach and intestines to keep them calm for several hours or until the condition corrects itself.

As is the case with all stomach remedies, you must first experiment by trying several of them to find which ones work most efficaciously for your own system, providing the needed cure without causing additional problems elsewhere in your system.

In the cases of insufficient and excessive elimination, by all means attempt first to balance your system in such away as to correct the problem naturally, by proper diet. What is right for one person may not, in the final analysis, be right for another. And if your system requires elimination only once a day, do not simply decide that this is insufficient and start taking laxatives to promote a twice-a-day elimination. The most ridiculous situation of all is to take an antidiarrheal medication to reduce the effect of diarrhea, then take a laxative a few hours later to promote elimination! We are, of course, a nation of pill-swallowers, but do try to apply a measure of reason.

Nausea

Nausea is another commonplace problem that can be corrected with medication, but again, nausea can be caused by any of a number of serious ailments that require a physician's attention.

Many of the seasick remedies or motion-sickness palliatives will act to reduce nausea and vomiting. The remedy, once taken, must stay down to be effective.

The products of nausea are an almost pure acid-like substance, welling up toward the throat. Frequently an ordinary antacid will reduce this to a level where it becomes tolerable. However, should vomiting occur, immediately wash the mouth with water to reduce the potency of the acidous products. These can cause not only a sour taste in the mouth, but can affect the tooth enamel and some of the sensitive mucous membranes in the mouth and throat as well.

Other Digestive Problems

Another problem, called "butterflies in the stomach," is the result of nervousness. Actors and actresses often suffer this problem just prior to going on stage and often try to correct it with alcohol — a big mistake! This problem, technically called "muscle tonus," is caused by our own natural instincts for survival. When we feel we are faced with threat or danger, the adrenalin flows rapidly into the stomach, causing this condition. It's good for you, too. It puts you on edge, makes all your senses their keenest, and you are as prepared as you can be for anything that might transpire. The condition is a vestigial one that goes back to our Cro-Magnon ancestors. You might feel these butterflies just before making a speech before a group of business associates. Your great-great-grandfather's ditto, back in the stone ages, felt it just prior to attacking a dinosaur! But whether it's a dinosaur or your boss, the cure is simple. Just hyperventilate by taking four or five very deep breaths. The condition will ease almost at once.

If there is one stomach problem that causes severe embarassment, and one that all of us are subject to at one time or another, it's flatulence. Stomach gases, passing out through the anus with a loud noise and accompanying foul odor. Usually when you sense that it's about to commence, you tighten the anal sphincter muscle and are quite uncomfortable. The one surest cure for this, of course, is to avoid gas-producing foods.

One place where this can be a real problem is — believe it or not — in flight! If the cabin of the plane is not properly pressurized, gases trapped in the stomach or intestine can expand and cause a great deal of pressure buildup, along with accompanying pain and discomfort.

To eliminate the problems of gas buildup, certain remedies are available over the counter for self-medication. These are usually coupled with other stomach distress medications and will serve to reduce gas.

One little-known remedy in this country is widely used in European countries as a specific. It is ordinary, chemically pure charcoal. In Europe, people brush their teeth with the black charcoal, for it is mildly abrasive. They then swallow the used dentifrice, for it "sweetens the stomach." How does charcoal work? It adsorbs the gas. Absorption is something else entirely. Adsorption is a process whereby the agent permits its surfaces to become coated with the material to be adsorbed, whereas absorption is a process in which the material is taken in. To expose additional surface area, modern charcoal is activated by treating it with steam under high pressure. The charcoal is then packed in capsules (it's also available in granular and tablet form) and is simply swallowed. When it reaches the stomach, it adsorbs excess gases and other discomfort-producing materials, including acids. It is also used as a specific for counteracting certain poisons and is used in drug overdoses. Interestingly enough, there are no counterindications for charcoal, but it should not be used where other medications are being taken. If you are taking aspirin, for example, do not take charcoal. The charcoal sees the aspirin as a foreign element and removes and eliminates it from the system. However, activated charcoal itself is perfectly safe for anybody to injest. While we are not specifically dealing with the matter here, you can buy activated charcoal in pellet form and mix this with pet foods. Your pet will have a cleaner, fresher breath as a result.

You can buy activated charcoal at any pharmacy. Again, and purely as an interesting sidelight, for it does deal with the stomach, one manufacturer of activated charcoal, The Requa Company, ran some tests a few years ago at Downstate Medical Center in New York. Hangover (upset stomach plus headache) is attributed to the congeners, or impurities, in many alcoholic beverages. Yet it is these same congeners that provide the bouquet and flavor of these drinks. Activated charcoal eliminates the congeners in your stomach, with the result that hangover is also eliminated. Before, during or after drinking, take one activated charcoal capsule for each ounce of liquor imbibed, and you won't have a problem the next morning. The congeners are present in all liquors except vodka, which is made by filtering through charcoal and possesses neither odor nor taste. Wines are particularly high in congeners.

If you do not happen to have activated charcoal on hand, simply toast a piece of bread until it is dark black, then eat this without any spread or butter. It works almost as well.

As with any other form of medication, always follow the dosage recommendations on the package and do not exceed these.

How important are the stomach remedies from a consumer point of view? Obviously, they're very important. Digestive aids and antacids were kicked off with advertising to you, the general public, with a total budget of almost $50 million in 1975. The advertising seems to have interested you, too. You spent $241,820,000 on laxatives alone, plus an additional $94,600,000 on diarrhea remedies!

The following pages contain excerpts adapted from the July-August 1974 issue of *FDA Consumer*. Any changes made in the text reflect only the passage of time.

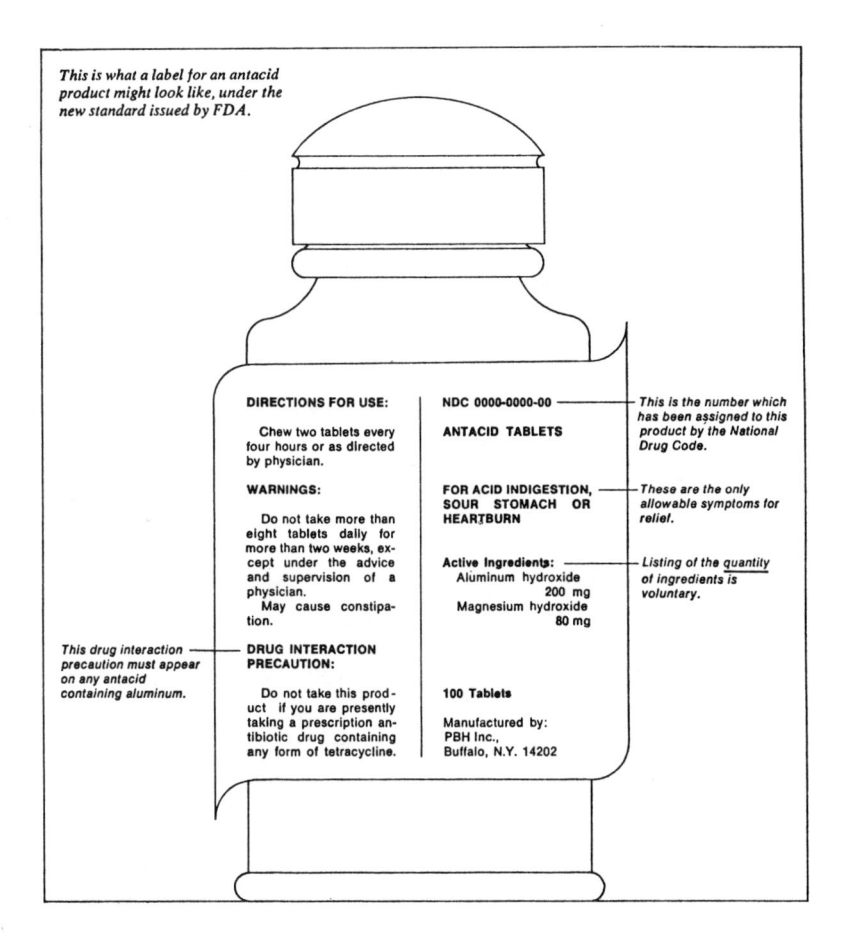

This is what a label for an antacid product might look like, under the new standard issued by FDA.

DIRECTIONS FOR USE:

Chew two tablets every four hours or as directed by physician.

WARNINGS:

Do not take more than eight tablets daily for more than two weeks, except under the advice and supervision of a physician.
May cause constipation.

This drug interaction precaution must appear on any antacid containing aluminum.

DRUG INTERACTION PRECAUTION:

Do not take this product if you are presently taking a prescription antibiotic drug containing any form of tetracycline.

NDC 0000-0000-00

ANTACID TABLETS

FOR ACID INDIGESTION, SOUR STOMACH OR HEARTBURN

Active Ingredients:
Aluminum hydroxide
200 mg
Magnesium hydroxide
80 mg

100 Tablets

Manufactured by:
PBH Inc.,
Buffalo, N.Y. 14202

This is the number which has been assigned to this product by the National Drug Code.

These are the only allowable symptoms for relief.

Listing of the quantity of ingredients is voluntary.

Antacids

When you pick up an antacid at your neighborhood pharmacy or supermarket, you're going to see some important changes on the label.

Gone are the claims that the antacid is safe and effective for a multitude of ills, from nervous stomach to hangover.

Gone are the many confusing formulations, each making its own special claims.

Instead, you will know that every antacid product you see is safe and effective and that all the information you need to use the product correctly is on the label.

For example, you will see only three therapeutic claims on antacid labels: that the product is safe and effective for the symptomatic relief of "heartburn," "sour stomach," and/or acid indigestion.

In addition, many antacids will have special warnings. And any antacid containing aluminum will warn consumers not to take the antacid while they are taking the prescription antibiotic tetracycline. Aluminum can reduce the effectiveness of tetracycline by preventing or reducing its absorption in the body.

More importantly, there will be only 13 acceptable ingredients or groups of ingredients, each of them proved safe and effective.

These important changes result from an order issued by the Food and Drug Administration June 4, 1974, which requires the manufacturers of all nonprescription antacid products to meet a new standard. The standard is the first issued under FDA's massive review of all nonprescription drugs.

Antacids continue to be sold in dosage forms to which consumers have become accustomed: chewable and non-chewable tablets, liquids, effervescent tablets or powder to be dissolved in water, and chewing gum with an antacid coating.

Labeling now provides information so that consumers can make meaningful comparisons between similar products and avoid those containing ingredients which they should not take.

For example, under the heading "Warning," the label must say: "Do not take more than (maximum recommended daily dosage, broken down by age groups if appropriate) in a 24-hour period, or use the maximum dosage of this product for more than 2 weeks, except under the advice and supervision of a physician."

Certain products must carry special warnings. For example, products that cause constipation in 5 percent or more of persons who take the maximum recommended dosage must warn: "May cause constipation." Also products that may cause laxation in 5 percent or more of the users must warn the consumer of such an effect.

Products containing relatively high amounts of magnesium, sodium, potassium, or lactose must also warn consumers. Magnesium or potassium should not be used by people with kidney disease, except on advice of a physician. Lactose should be avoided by people allergic to milk, and sodium should be avoided by those on a sodium-restricted diet.

Any company that wants to market an antacid that deviates from this standard must seek FDA approval.

The new standard affects about 8,000 currently marketed antacid products. In 1972, antacid sales were estimated at $117 million.

All products must have conformed to the new standard by June 4, 1975. New labeling requirements for products promoted only to doctors were to be provided by June 4, 1976. This professional labeling must include information about the capacity of the product to neutralize stomach acid.

Publication of the final order setting this new standard for antacids concluded one of the most intensive scientific reviews ever undertaken by a regulatory agency. For nearly a year, beginning in May 1972, seven of the Nation's leading experts in gastrointestinal theraphy, pharmacists, and pharmacologists focused their attention on all available evidence on antacids.

FDA's library performed a search of all recent antacid literature, and more than 50 companies who market antacids provided enough data to fill a shelf 12 feet long. The panel members met six times for 2 or 3 days at a time, and received information at each meeting from any interested party who wished to appear and present information.

In addition, the panel consisted of two nonvoting members representing consumer groups and industry. They participated in every meeting. Their function was to assure public awareness of and participation in the Government's decision-making process.

This entire process resulted in a report and a proposed new standard to assure the safety and effectiveness of antacids. FDA allowed opportunities at several stages for consumers and industry to comment on the proposed standard, and held a hearing January 21, 1974, to receive further information and comments.

The final order June 4 was the first issued as part of FDA's class-by-class review of all OTC drugs. (The process by which this review is being conducted was described in "OTC Drug Review: An Update," FDA CONSUMER, May 1974.)

Commissioner Schmidt hailed the action as a "significant milestone in FDA's attempt to establish a more manageable system for assuring safe and effective formulas and full labeling for all the hundreds of thousands of nonprescription drugs on the market."

The same process followed by FDA for antacids will be followed for the other 26 classes of OTC drugs. It will be several years before final orders are issued for all the classes.

When they are, the public will have greater assurance that every OTC drug available is not only safe and effective, but is properly labeled and formulated. The new standards also will result in changes in advertising claims, which are regulated by the Federal Trade Commission. Several firms have already modified their television advertising and their product ingredients, even before the official standards were issued.

The day after the antacid standard was published, Dr. Schmidt discussed it in testimony before the Senate Monopoly Subcommittee. Dr. Schmidt cited four significant aspects of the standard:

- That each antacid product must not only be composed of safe and effective ingredients, but that the effectiveness of the finished product must be confirmed by meeting an acid neutralizing test developed by the expert panel.

- That the indications for the use of antacids should be limited to those conditions clearly related to excess acid in the stomach, and should therefore exclude vague or unsubstantiated claims that now appear on many antacid labels.

- That cautionary and warning statements should be concise and readily understandable.

- That combinations of antacids and other drugs should not be permitted where evidence is lacking that each ingredient contributes to the claimed effect or effects and where there is no specific group of people to which the claims apply.

In testifying before the Senate subcommittee, Dr. Schmidt stated his view that the standard issued by FDA has the force and effect of law. Some people claim that the standard should be only guidelines for industry to follow.

Because antacids were the first class of OTC drugs considered by FDA as part of its overall review, a number of broader issues applying to all OTC drugs were raised which were decided by the Commissioner.

Perhaps the most highly publicized issue was that regarding the combination of an antacid and a salicylate (aspirin). The best example of this is Alka-Seltzer.

Opponents of the combination of an antacid and a salicylate maintained that it is irrational and unsafe because antacids are designed to relieve acid indigestion, while salicylates can cause bleeding in the stomach.

In his testimony June 5, Dr. Schmidt pointed out that the combination is indeed irrational — for use solely as an antacid.

But, the Commissioner added, the combination does conform to FDA's policy regarding combination drugs, "in that both ingredients are indicated and effective for the concurrent symptoms of acid indigestion and headache." The Commissioner agreed there are people who have both symptoms at the same time.

Therefore, the Commissioner concluded that combinations of antacids with salicylates may continue, with proper formulation and labeling.

The Commissioner noted that the use of salicylates is being reviewed by the Panel on Internal Analgesics, which will recommend to the Agency acceptable conditions for use for pain relievers, including their concurrent use with antacids.

In deciding the antacid-salicylate issue, the Commissioner expressed the view that nonprescription drugs composed of two or more ingredients can still be marketed, provided that there is a reason for combining the ingredients, and that the consumer is not exposed to an unreasonable risk.

The Commissioner concluded, however, that adding an anticholinergic ingredient (which decreases stomach activity) to an OTC antacid would not be permitted. Also rejected were products that combine an antacid with a laxative, an enzyme, or an antiemetic (which decreases nausea). None of these uses constitutes rational therapy, the Commissioner found.

A second issue related to the warning on OTC drug labels to keep drugs out of the reach of children. The Commissioner decided to modify the present warning and require that the following statement appear on drug labels:

> *"Keep this and all drugs out of the reach of children. In case of accidental overdose, seek professional assistance or contact your poison control center immediately."*

A third issue related to the inclusion on the label of the statement concerning possible drug interactions. Pharmacy groups testified at the January 21 hearing that the label should tell the consumer to consult his pharmacist as well as his physician in case of a possible interaction.

The Commissioner resolved this issue by requiring that the label include a separate section headed "Drug Interaction Precautions," which will state the interaction problem involved with a particular OTC drug. For the first time, the consumer can learn from the label that he should not take the product while also taking a particular prescription drug. The drug interaction precaution for all aluminum-containing OTC antacid products is the first one to be required. Other precautions will be required for other OTC drugs, that may interact with prescription drugs.

In announcing this decision, the Commissioner said:

"The purpose of OTC medication is to permit consumers to engage in self-medication without medical or other professional supervision, or in any event with the least amount of supervision feasible. Directing that consumers consult health professionals of any type would seem appropriate only if it is concluded that this is the only possible method of assuring the safe and effective use of the drug.

"Accordingly, although the Commissioner recognizes the availablity of useful drug information through all health professionals, he concluded that it is unnecessary and inappropriate that they be designated on the label in any manner with respect to this particular matter in view of the availability of fully informative labeling which obviates such reference."

The OTC drug review which generated the antacid standard and these more general issues is based on the 1962 Drug Amendments to the Food, Drug, and Cosmetic Act, which required for the first time that all drugs be proven effective as well as safe.

FDA then undertook to review for effectiveness all drugs for which marketing applications had been submitted since 1938, when the safety requirement was added to the drug law. That review disclosed that very few OTC drugs had been the subjects of applications. The initial review, therefore, was limited to prescription drugs.

In 1972, FDA launched the present review to consider 27 categories of OTC drugs and set standards comparable to those now set for antacids.

FDA is using advisory committees as primary sources for this review. In his June 5 testimony, Dr. Schmidt said: "To enable us to make the best possible judgments, we have and will continue to use advisory committees to provide us with information, interpretation, and advice which will supplement that generated internally. . . . The functions of the over-the-counter drug panels demonstrates the increasingly important role of broadly constituted scientific advisory bodies as integral parts of our regulatory process."

In announcing the antacid standard, Dr. Schmidt also reaffirmed FDA's commitment to a system of self-medication in this country. "Self-medication is an essential part of our health care system. Fundamental to self-medication is the requirement that any drug available for use at the purchaser's own initiative must be safe and effective for its intended purpose.

"It is of equal importance that any such drug must be fully labeled and fairly advertised so that an individual can indeed medicate himself for appropriate conditions safely and effectively, without professional supervision."

"I submit that the publication of our first over-the-counter monograph represents a significant milestone toward this goal."

Acceptable Ingredients

The new standard for over-the-counter antacid products recognizes 13 acceptable active ingredients. They are:

- Aluminum-containing ingredients
- Bicarbonate-containing ingredients
- Bismuth-containing ingredients
- Calcium-containing ingredients

- Citrate-containing ingredients
- Magnesium-containing ingredients
- Phosphate-containing ingredients
- Potassium-containing ingredients
- Sodium-containing ingredients
- Tartrate-containing ingredients
- Sodium bicarbonate
- Glycine (aminoacetic acid)
- Dried milk solids

In addition, in a different standard for antiflatulent products, simethicone with a maximum daily dose of 500 milligrams is permitted in a product labeled "to alleviate or relieve the symptoms of gas."

Charles R. Beek is a freelance writer on medical topics, and in a recent issue of the *FDA Consumer,* he commented on laxatives. We felt that his pertinent statements were well-worth repeating here.

Laxatives: What Does 'Regular' Mean?

Television commercials tell us that for good health and well-being we should all be "regular." We needn't be troubled with "irregularity," biliousness, aftermeal discomfort or headaches, if we will take the named laxative. Even Mae West of early film fame attributes the longevity of her good looks to a daily enema.

An independent panel of physicians, pharmacologists, and consultants appointed by FDA to review the safety, effectiveness, and labeling of over-the-counter (OTC) laxatives has found nevertheless that what the public knows about regular or normal bowel functioning still leaves a great deal to be desired. The Advisory Review Panel on OTC Laxatives, Antidiarrheal, Emetic, and Antiemetic Drug Products, said:

"In the United States, preoccupation with the bowel seems to be the concern of a significant proportion of our population judging from the inordinately large number of laxative agents available and by the significant expenditure for OTC laxatives. The Panel is of the opinion that a large segment of the population is not only 'bowel-conscious,' but also has many misconceptions of normal bowel function. The laity is under the impression that serious and health endangering consequences will occur if the bowel is not evacuated daily. The Panel is of the opinion that there is widespread overuse of self-prescribed laxatives. Extensive advertising by the pharmaceutical industry has contributed to this problem."

This report is the first step toward setting definitive Federal standards for OTC laxative, anti-diarrheal, emetic, and antiemetic drug products, comparable to those now set for antacids. The final antacid standards, established June 4, 1974, were the first issued as part of the massive class-by-class review launched by FDA in 1972 to evaluate all OTC drugs. (How the review was being conducted was described in "OTC Drug Review: An Update," *FDA Consumer,* May 1974.) The laxative, antidiarrheal, emetic, and antiemetic class is the third of 27 groups of OTC drugs to be reviewed.

FDA's final standards describe conditions under which OTC laxative, antidiarrheal, emetic, and antiemetic products will be recognized as safe and effective and not misbranded. They will include the specific active ingredients, combinations of active ingredients, combination criteria, and labeling statements that will be allowed on marketed products.

Any company that markets an OTC laxative, antidiarrheal, antiemetic, or emetic product will have to use only those ingredients found to be acceptable. Labeling will have to conform to the requirements set forth in the standards. Any company wanting to market a product that deviates from the standards either will have to petition the Commissioner of Food and Drugs to amend the standards or get approval through FDA's New Drug Application procedures.

The Panel's findings on laxative ingredients and labeling in marketed products are set out in three categories:

• Ingredients generally recognized as safe and effective and as not mislabeled. The Panel recommends that ingredients and labeling in this category be included in the final standards.

• Ingredients not generally recognized as safe and effective or which are mislabeled. The Panel recommends that such ingredients be eliminated or the labeling claims corrected within 6 months after publication of the final standards in the *Federal Register*. This would be required regardless of whether testing is undertaken to justify their future use.

• Ingredients or labeling claims for which the available data are insufficient to permit final classification at this time. The Panel recommends that ingredients or labeling claims in this category be permitted to remain in use for 2 years after the date of publication of the final standards in the *Federal Register*, if the manufacturer or distributor of any such drug conducts tests and studies during that period to satisfy the questions raised by the Panel.

Although the Advisory Panel's report did not impose any legal requirements on the pharmaceutical industry at this time, it does provide much useful information for the industry and the consuming public. It can help consumers select the right type of laxative product for a particular indication or problem, and it can help manufacturers determine whether changes may be necessary in formulations or labeling or whether additional supporting data may be required for continued use of questioned ingredients or claims.

The Panel took issue with a number of advertising claims that often are heard in connection with laxatives. "Any statement that suggests a laxative is somehow 'natural' because of its source is misleading," the Panel said, "because it implies that the product or ingredient is a 'natural way' to induce laxation. It is not considered natural to take any laxative."

"Irregularity" as an indication for use of laxatives also is misleading, the Panel said, because "regularity" of bowel movement is not essential to health or well-being. Variability of frequency of bowel movements is normal within certain limits, the Panel found. Based on two recent studies, normal limits for bowel habits were suggested. In one study of 1,055 industrial workers (655 women and 400 men) in the London area, it was found that bowel movements ranging from three a week to three a day can be normal. In the other study, involving 115 healty adult men in a U.S. Federal correction institution, the interval between stools varied from 9 to 57 hours.

The Panel said that the bowel habits of many laxative users seem to fall within the normal range, and these people apparently have no physical or organic condition requiring the use of laxatives. Simple constipation most often results from improper diet, inadequate fluid intake, insufficient exercise, or a change of habits due to travel, the Panel said. There are only a few valid indications for the use of laxatives, according to the Panel, and "relief for simple constipation often may be achieved by proper diet, including foods with adequate fiber content, adequate fluid intake, and the prompt response to the urge to evacuate the bowels."

The Panel recommended a number of specific changes in current labeling so consumers can compare products and get a better understanding of how they work. This would enable consumers to avoid products containing ingredients they should not take. For example, the Panel has recommended that all laxative labels state that the product should be used only "for the short-term relief of constipation." To help the consumer know what to expect from taking the product, the Panel recommended that the labels also include the specific mode by which the product acts to relieve constipation: "To increase frequency of bowel movements," "To soften stool," or "To increase bulk of the stool."

The Panel also called for a label warning to consumers on products containing relatively high amounts of sodium. It recommends requiring a sodium statement of content per dosage unit where sodium exceeds 23 milligrams per maximum daily dose. If sodium exceeds 345 milligrams per daily dose, the Panel said, the label should warn against use of the product by people on a low salt diet or by those who have kidney disease "except under the advice and supervision of a physician."

For stimulant-type laxatives, the Panel suggested the following label warning: "Prolonged or continued use of this product can lead to laxative dependency and loss of normal bowel function. Serious side effects from prolonged use or overdose can occur. This product should be used only occasionally, but, in any event no longer than daily for 1 week, except on the advice of a physician."

Castor oil, a long-familiar laxative ingredient, should be taken infrequently and then only as a one-time, single dose, the Panel warned.

The Panel divided laxatives into broad categories, based on how they are supposed to work. The categories and modes of action are:

• Bulk-forming laxative: Promotes evacuation of the bowel by increasing bulk volume and water content of the stools.

• Stimulant laxative: Promotes bowel movement by one or more direct actions on the intestine.

• Hyperosmotic and saline laxatives: The hyperosmotic agent attracts water into the stool. The saline agent increases water in the intestine, thereby promoting bowel movement.

• Lubricant and stool softener laxatives: Lubricant agents lubricate the contents of the intestinal tract, promoting easier bowel movements. Stool softeners penetrate and soften the stool.

For all of these laxative categories, the Panel recommended only 25 acceptable ingredients, or groups of ingredients, as proved safe and effective.

Six of these ingredients are used in bulk-forming laxatives, which the Panel found are among the safest of laxatives. Bulk-forming laxatives generally are not absorbed from the digestive tract and therefore would have less possibility of causing any adverse side effects, the Panel pointed out. It also noted, however, that most of these laxatives should be taken with a full glass of liquid to minimize the risk of digestive tract obstruction.

Eight stimulant-type laxative ingredients were found safe and effective, but the Panel cautioned that this type of laxative should be used only occasionally. It is possible for an ingredient to be found generally safe and effective, while specific labeling claims made in its behalf are questionable. This was the case with dehydrocholic acid. The Panel approved it as a stimulant-type laxative ingredient, but found unacceptable the claims that it relieves "indigestion," "excessive belching," "aftermeal discomfort," or "the sensation of abdominal fullness."

Four saline and two hyperosmotic laxative ingredients were found safe and effective. The Panel recommended that saline laxatives be restricted to occasional use, because serious saline imbalances have been reported with their long-term daily use. It also urged that products containing glycerin — one of the two acceptable hyperosmotic ingredients — should state: Glycerin administered rectally may produce in some individuals rectal discomfort or a burning sensation."

Two lubricant ingredients, plain mineral oil and emulsified mineral oil, and three stool softener ingredients were considered acceptable by the Panel. The Panel concluded that these products as well as all laxatives should not be used for a period longer than 1 week except under the advice and supervision of a physician.

Mineral oil preparations are required to have a warning against use in conjunction with a stool softener. In addition, plain mineral oil would be labeled for use only at bedtime and not for use in certain individuals — including infants, pregnant women, and bedridden or aged patients — except under advice and supervision of a physician. Emulsified mineral oil would be labeled for divided doses, the first dose on rising and the second dose taken only at bedtime and neither dose at mealtimes.

The Panel also found that dioctyl sulfosuccinate preparations (one form of the acceptable stool softener) might increase the potency of other drugs being taken and recommended that the label should state: "Drug interaction precaution: Do not take this product if you are presently taking a prescription drug or mineral oil." The Panel also concluded that rectal suppositories which release carbon dioxide are safe and effective as an aid in evacuation of the bowel.

The complete list of laxative ingredients found safe and effective by the Panel is as follows:

- Bulk-forming laxatives: Dietary bran, cellulose derivatives, karaya, malt soup extract, polycarbophil, psyllium preparations.
- Stimulant laxatives: Aloe, bisacodyl, cascara sagrada preparations, castor oil, danthron, dehydrocholic acid, phenolphthalein, senna preparations.
- Saline laxatives: Magnesium citrate, magnesium hydroxide, magnesium sulfate, phosphate preparations.
- Hyperosmotic laxatives: Glycerin, sorbitol.
- Lubricant laxatives: Plain mineral oil and emulsified mineral oil.
- Stool softener laxatives: Sulfosuccinate preparations.
- Miscellaneous laxative: Released carbon dioxide from combined sodium biphosphate anhydrous, sodium acid pyrophosphate, and sodium bicarbonate.

In addition to laxatives, the Panel also reviewed over-the-counter drugs to control diarrhea (antidiarrheals). The Panel defined diarrhea as the abnormally frequent passage of watery stools, self-limiting (24-48 hours), usually with no identifiable cause. The main factor contributing to diarrhea is the excess water. Diarrhea unassociated with fever or blood in the stool, but sometimes associated with symptoms such as loss of appetite, abdominal cramps, nausea and vomiting is common. The Panel further noted that antidiarrheals provide only symptomatic relief and are most effective in the mildest types of diarrhea. For the antidiarrheal products, the Panel found only two active ingredients or groups of active ingredients acceptable. These are opiates, including opium powder, tincture of opium, and paregoric; and polycarbophil.

The Panel also reviewed OTC products to induce vomiting (emetics) or prevent it (antiemetics). Although the Panel received no submission of emetics from the pharmaceutical industry or other sources, it elected to review ipecac syrup as an OTC emetic drug to induce vomiting (emesis) in case of poisoning. It concluded that ipecac syrup is safe and effective for such an emergency when used in the recommended dose of 15 milliliters (½ oz.) in persons above 1 year of age and a dose of 5 to a maximum of 10 milliliters (1 to 2 teaspoonfuls) in infants under 1 year old. OTC product containers are limited to not more than 30 milliliters (1 oz.) of ipecac syrup. The labeling recommended by the Panel also would warn against use if strychnine, corrosives such as alkalies (lyes) and strong acids, or petroleum distillates such as kerosene, gasoline, paint thinner, or cleaning fluid have been ingested.

Of the antiemetics reviewed, only two ingredients or groups of ingredients were found generally safe and effective. These are benzhydryl piperazine antihistamines, including cyclizine and meclizine, and dimenhydrinate. The Panel warned, however, that all OTC antiemetics should be used only in cases of nausea due to motion sickness. There was insufficient information to determine if these drugs are effective in the treatment of nausea due to "indigestion, upset stomach, or fullness."

The Panel concluded that insufficient evidence exists to determine the role of certain ingredients used in laxative, antidiarrheal, emetic, and antiemetic products. It proposed that these products continue to be sold on the market for 2 years after the final standard adopted by the FDA is published, if the manufacturer or distributor promptly undertakes testing to satisfy the questions raised by the Panel.

There are 13 laxative indgredients in this category. They are agar, bran tablets, carrangeenan, guar gum, aloin, bile salts and ox bile, d-calcium pantothenate, frangula, prune concentrate dehydrate and prune powder, Chinese rhubarb, sodium oleate, tartaric acid and tartrate preparations, and poloxalkol.

The active ingredients in the antidiarrheal products group that require more study, the Panel said, are attapulgite activated, charcoal activated, kaolin, pectin, atropine sulfate, homatropine methylbromide, hyoscyamine sulfate, alumina powder, bismuth salts, calcium hydroxide, phenyl salicylate, zinc phenolsufonate, calcium carbonate, *Lactobacilli acidophillus* and *bulgaricus,* and sodium carboxymethylcellulose.

The Panel found four ingredients in the antiemetic group, bismuth subsalicylate, phenyl salicylate, phosphorated carbohydrate, and zinc phenolsulfonate, that require more study. The review is still under way.

Publication of the Panel report completes an intensive scientific review effort that began in April 1973, when the Advisory Panel convened its first meeting. Two months earlier FDA had issued a notice in the *Federal Register* requesting data and information on all laxative, antidiarrheal, emetic, and antiemetic active ingredients in drug products. Panel members met 12 times through January 1975, for 2 days at a time.

Over 40 firms submitted information on over 130 of their products containing over 100 different labeled ingredients. In addition, the FDA library performed a search of all recent literature on laxative, antidiarrheal, emetic, and antiemetic products. The Panel reviewed the literature, the various data submissions, and listened to testimony from all interested parties who expressed a desire to appear.

In addition to the seven voting members appointed by the Commissioner of Food and Drugs, four nonvoting liaison representatives of consumer groups and industry served on the Panel. FDA provided administrative support to the Panel.

ANTACIDS

Product	Form	Calcium Carbonate	Aluminum Hydroxide	Magnesium Oxide or Hydroxide	Magnesium Trisylicate	Other	Sodium Content
Alka-2 (Miles)	chewable tablet	500 mg					
Alka-Seltzer (Miles)	effervescent tablet	780 mg				sodium bicarbonate, 1.008 g potassium bicarbonate 300 mg citric acid 800 mg	
BiSoDol (Whitehall)	tablet, powder	195 mg (tablet)		180 mg (tablet)		sodium bicarbonate (powder), magnesium carbonate (powder), peppermint oil (tablet, powder)	0.036 mg/tablet 157 mg/tsp powder
Chooz (Plough)	gum tablet	360 mg			268 mg		
Di-Gel (Plough)	tablet, suspension		codried with magnesium carbonate, 282 mg/tablet	85 mg/tab 87 mg/5 ml		simethicone 25 mg/tablet or 5 ml	10.6 mg/tablet 8.5 mg/5 ml

Gelusil (Warner-Chilcott)	tablet, suspension	250 mg/tablet or 5 ml		500 mg/tab or 5 ml	mint flavor		9 mg/tab 8 mg/5 ml
Maalox (Rorer)	suspension	225 mg/5 ml	200 mg/5 ml				2.5 mg/5 ml
Mylanta (Stuart)	tablet, suspension	200 mg/tab or 5 ml	200 mg/tab or 5 ml		simethicone 20 mg/tab or 5 ml		0.79 mg/tab 11.7 mg/5 ml
Nutrajel (Cenci)	suspension	300 mg/5 ml					
Phillips Milk of Magnesia (Glenbrook)	suspension, tablet		2.27-2.62 g/ 30 ml 311 mg/tab		peppermint oil, 1,166 mg 30 ml or tab		
Rolaids (Warner-Lambert)	tablet				dihydroxy-aluminum sodium carbonate, 334 mg		53 mg
Titralac (Riker)	tablet, suspension	420 mg/ tab, 1 g/ 5 ml			glycine, 180 mg/ tablet, 300 mg/ 5 ml		11 mg/5 ml
Tums (Lewis-Howe)	tablet	500 mg			peppermint oil		2.7 mg

LAXATIVES

Product (Manufacturer)	Form	Stimulant	Bulk Forming	Emollient/Lubricant	Other Laxatives	Other Ingredients
Carter's Little Pills (Carter)	tablet	aloe, 16 mg podophyllum 4.0 mg				
Correctol (Plough)	tablet	yellow phenolphthalein 64.8 mg		dioctyl sodium sulfosuccinate, 100 mg		
Ex-Lax (Ex-Lax)	chocolate tablet	yellow phenolphthalein 90 mg				
Feen-A-Mint (Plough)	chewing gum chewable tab mint	yellow phenolphthalein 97.2 mg				
Fletcher's Castoria (Glenbrook)	liquid	senna, 6.5%				
Haley's M-O (Glenbrook)	emulsion			mineral oil, 25%	magnesium hydroxide, 75%	

Metamucil (Searle)	powder	psyllium mucilloid 50%	dextrose, 50%
Nature's Remedy (Lewis-Howe)	tablet		aloe, 143 mg cascara sagrada, 127 mg
Phillips Milk of Magnesia (Glenbrook)	suspension tablet		magnesium hydroxide 2.27-2.62 g /30 ml, 311 mg tablet	peppermint oil, 1.166 mg/30 ml or tablet
Sal Hepatica (Bristol-Myers)	granules			sodium phosphate, sodium bicarbonate, citric acid, anhydrous sodium citrate, tribasic sodium citrate dibasic
Saraka (Plough)	granules	karaya gum	frangula
Serutan (J.B. Williams)	powder granules	psyllium 100%	

Chapter Eighteen

Muscle Problems

Muscles are the tissues that expand and contract at will to move the limbs to which they are connected. All bodily movement is actuated by muscles; if they are properly treated they can do all the work they have to do, and do it well. Improperly treated, muscles will rebel and cause problems. Muscles, you see, must be developed and built up to do the work that is required of them. If you lead a relatively sedentary existence and a group of friends suggest a ski weekend, that's all well and good. But your muscles may not be ready for violent physical exertion, and this sudden onslaught of activity and exercise can result in, at the very least, severe cramping. The man who skis regularly has already brought his muscles to a proper tone and may not have that problem.

Before you attempt to call on your muscles for extra work, build up to the level of that work very slowly, stretching and exercising the muscles so they can handle the work you plan to call on them for.

The muscles are connected to the bone by tendons or ligaments. These are simply tough pieces of tissue that tie the working muscle to the bone it must move. Sometimes, as in so many other cases, you might attempt to minister to yourself and treat a torn muscle or ligament as if it were a simple cramp. While you might not be doing any actual damage, you are delaying a visit to a physician. Sometimes such tears require complete immobilization while the body heals itself, and sometimes surgery might be required to make proper restoration. The torn muscle or ligament is not something that you should self-medicate!

Cramp or spasm, however, is another thing entirely. An overworked muscle "locks up" and notifies you through extreme pain that something is wrong.

This can happen to athletes as well as to the most deskbound of people! The work a muscle is called on for is relative. The athlete who dredges the last bit of strength during a race can get a cramp. The sedentary person can get the same kind of cramp simply by bending over. Often after a good work-out you may suddenly be stricken with a cramp in the calf muscle in the middle of the night. You wake up with a severe pain. The best way to relieve this sort of pain is to fully extend the afflicted limb and stand on the leg with all your weight. This will be even more painful for a moment until the muscle relaxes. Then the pain will pass. It will help to knead the muscle strongly for a time until relief is felt, as this will help the muscle to relax.

Once the spasm has passed, the muscle should be allowed to rest for a time before it is exercised again. Since the cramp comes on suddenly, this is likely to be a bit unsettling to the entire bodily system. A sharp pain is a frightening thing, especially if it comes in the middle of the night. Administer two aspirins for a calming effect. And if violent exercise must be repeated, build up to it slowly.

People who regularly indulge in violent physical activity will always undergo a "warm-up" before participating in such activity. *Karate-ka,* students of the martial arts, call upon their bodies for the most strenuous violent physical activity known to man. They always begin with class exercises to ascertain that their bodies are supple and ready to fight. They attend classes regularly, practicing *kata,* or drills so that when an emergency does take place, they are well prepared to meet it.

Muscle trauma can also cause spasm, and the karate student uses this as a tool as well. Strike a muscle violently from outside, and it will go into spasm and lock up. We've seen karate experts take advantage of this by forming what is called a "knife hand" and, by striking an opponent's muscles, cause spasm and bind the man so he is totally immobilized by his own muscles.

Should you avoid violent physical exercise? Not at all. Doctors recommend a program of physical exertion, for your heart is a muscle too, and keeping it in good condition can help you to a longer, more fruitful life. A program of regular exercise is to be recommended, and this can take the form of jogging or running, handball, basketball, or regular workouts at a gymnasium. Our grandfathers used to go to the local sandlot and play baseball on a Sunday afternoon. Today we're content to watch a baseball game on television. The exercise you get by watching is *not* the same!

What can — and should — you do when a muscle cramps up? Even if cramps do not occur, muscles that have been overworked can become sore and tired.

For a cramp, extend the limb so that the muscle is in full extension. This should immediately relieve the pain. Knead the muscle to help relax it and apply external heat in the form of a heating pad or hot water bottle wrapped in a towel. Allow the muscle to relax until it has fully recovered. Do not attempt to repeat or continue the exercise immediately after the pain has passed, or certainly it will return.

There are OTC medications that can be of great benefit when muscles become sore and tender. But your physician can prescribe muscle relaxants that are even faster acting and more beneficial. If you have a cardiac problem, muscle relaxants are usually contraindicated, and your physician should be told of such a problem before a prescription is written out.

Several rub-in ointments are available over the counter that can bring soothing relief. These are available either as ointments that are absorbed into the skin or as rub-on liquids. These operate in two ways. They contain counterirritants which are absorbed and help relieve surface pain, and they may contain in addition exothermic chemicals that generate heat. The chemicals cause blood to flow near the surface and you may even notice a reddening of the skin color where the chemicals have been applied. The flowing blood and the exothermic reaction of the chemicals create a feeling of warmth, which is soothing and comforting. The rubbing action as the chemical is applied also is soothing and relieving.

The chances are that when a muscle spasm strikes, you'll be able to do something about it, even if all you do is sit down and relax for awhile until the spasm passes. Unfortunately, you can't always do that easily. If you're swimming and get a cramp, the important thing is to avoid panic. Simply tread water and massage the cramped member until the cramp passes.

If you're operating machinery, simply do the best that you can. If you're tending a machine, turn it off until you can attend to it properly again. If you are in a moving vehicle, pull it over to the side and park, then take care of the cramp.

Where muscles seem to give way to cramp too quickly and too easily, the indications are that the muscles may require building up. However, simply to assume that this is cramp and nothing more is dead wrong. There are many muscle diseases that can result in serious bodily problems. When any problem manifests itself chronically, a smart move will be a visit to a physician for his diagnosis. To simply brush such problems off as "temporary" can be a costly error.

The muscles are the prime movers of the body and its component parts. Muscles receive stimulating information from the brain via the nervous system. If muscles do not act and react properly, the obvious answer — muscle problems — might not be the correct answer. Some measure of common sense is required before self-medication can be used.

If you have been reasonably sedentary and then, after a bout of severe (or relatively severe) exercise, you develop tiredness or a cramp which quickly responds to an analgesic rub and then disappears, chances are that the self-medication did indeed solve the problem.

If, however, the problem does not seem to be relieved after a suitable time, or if the muscle problem is one that may not seem to occur for any specific reason, see a physician.

Involuntary muscle action is another thing that frightens many people, and this can take several forms. You may develop a twitching of a leg muscle with no action on your part. Ordinarily this is no serious matter unless it occurs chronically. If it does, see your physician, who will no doubt recommend a series of tests and examinations to pinpoint and correct the cause of such a problem, which is usually nervous in origin.

The most important lessons to be learned in any discussion of muscular problems are: a) do not panic over them, b) by all means see a physician where even the remotest question about the problem exists, and c) depending on the nature and cause (if known) of the problem, you can attempt self-medication with the understanding that if the problem does not respond a physician will be consulted.

Chapter Nineteen

The Portable Medicine Cabinet

Our society is a highly mobile one. Everyone owns a car, we take vacation trips away from home, we're constantly on the go. We seem actually to live from trip to trip, and thanks to modern science, our transportation facilities have evolved to a highly refined degree that gives us the wherewithal to travel almost freely and unencumbered. You can reach into your wallet, extract a plastic credit card and then hop down to the airport. A scant few hours later, you can be dining in Europe. In less than two thousand years man has achieved a level of mobility that is, to say the least, wondrous! The airplane, that magic flying carpet that with jet power will whisk you to a foreign land in less than five hours, was invented only 60 years ago!

But we still have our health problems that go along with us wherever we travel. Should you visit a foreign country, it is usually no great problem, for most of the civilized countries of the world have more-than-adequate physicians who can treat you and prescribe. Their choices of self-medications are as wide as ours are, and the chances are that you'll see very familiar looking bottles on a pharmacist's shelf. They often sell the same brands as we have here. The language printed on the label might be different, but you'll see the same familiar label designs, and questioning will reveal that the products are the very same.

Even so, it's a wise idea to travel well prepared for emergencies.

When you think in terms of preparing a "portable medicine cabinet," chances are that your first attention will be directed toward first aid. However, you will want to include other items to meet your medical requirements while away from home.

The first thing to consider is how long you plan to be away and then add an extra supply that will carry you in case of emergency. After all, your plans can change. A plane might be delayed. You might elect to come back by boat instead. The boss might wire you to take a side trip while you're out there, and if you are taking regular medication, it would be foolish to take just exactly enough for the planned duration of your stay. This is especially true in the case of prescribed medication.

If you do not have sufficient supplies on hand, check with your physician and explain about your journey so that he can prescribe additional medication.

Where do you pack this portable medicine cabinet? This must go along with carry-on luggage, where it will always be accessible to you. It's sheer foolishness and lack of foresight to be served a meal on a plane and then remember that the pills you must take with that meal are stowed someplace beneath you in the luggage compartment. On steamships, it is also a procedure to stow heavy trunks and suitcases in the hold, where they will be inaccessible until the end of the voyage, which might last several days.

We like to prepare a traveling medicine cabinet using a lady's cosmetics case, which seems to be precisely the right size. We begin with a standard, commercially available first aid kit that will contain all of the requirements for emergencies. This goes into the case first, in one corner.

Next, we add the bottles and vials of all of the family's necessary prescription medications, each clearly and plainly marked with the family member's name and the dosage. We add a blob of color to the cap, assigning each family member a color of his own so that, with the case open and looking down at the top, we can quickly and easily spot the medications that each family member needs. The colors we use are the ones made for painting plastic airplane models. These same colors can be used to identify each family member's suitcase as well. In fact, in our own family, Josh even purchased a red cap so that the color coding would be complete. No need to tell you what his nickname got to be for the entire trip, either!

With the medications in place and the first aid kit installed, we next consider the specific needs of family members as far as non-prescription medications and vitamins are concerned. These are listed on paper, inspected to be sure the quantity is sufficient for the duration of the journey, plus an added amount just in case, and then checked off as they are placed in the kit.

Are we finished yet? Not half, we aren't. The medicines are now individually packed in plastic bags in case of moisture that had not been planned for, and this kit is then put in a large plastic bag and placed with other luggage that will be close at hand when it's needed.

Not everything goes into this kit, however. Certain items are Mom's responsibility. Any traveling that's done with youngsters is going to require a supply of Dramamine or some other motion-sickness remedy, and this goes into Mom's purse, along with aspirin and some hard candies, just in case. Dad's antacids are placed in his own shirt pocket where they will be handy.

What, exactly, should you take? It depends on where you're going and for how long. If it's simply a day's junket in the family car, you needn't load up as though it were a two-week's stay at the seashore. A bit of thoughtful application is required, and no single list can possibly cover every family's requirements. However, a good basic rule of thumb is to set aside one special container for medications of all sorts, and to know where that container is.

We've found that it's a good idea to buy the smallest-size containers of those nonprescription drug items that we use regularly. This may sound like a dichotomy, but it truly isn't. We also obtain the large economy size, and when we travel, the small vial, properly labeled, is refilled from the larger one. The small one goes on the trip with us, the large one remains at home.

We like to carry with us a headache remedy, an antacid, toothache drops, a suitable sunburn preventive and, if that's forgotten until too late, a sunburn cure. We take along the necessary motion sickness remedies, vitamins and eyedrops, all on a "just-in-case" basis.

A word of warning is required here.

We do not mean you to load yourself up like an ambulatory drugstore before you make a trip. The airlines will charge you for overweight luggage. Remember that unless you're headed for Tierra del Fuego at the bottom of the civilized world, chances are that you'll easily find a skilled physician and an ample source of medication. While you should take along those things that you may not be able to buy in a foreign country, the chances are that the other items you need will be available to you during your travels.

If you have prescription items you must take, we suggest you have the prescriptions refilled before traveling — even if you plan to travel only to another state. We've had the experience of having a pharmacist in Chicago refuse to fill a prescription we received in New York.

The same thing may apply to nonprescription drug items. The things that are available and commonplace in your home state may not be so readily available in foreign areas. We already know that Laetrile, for example, is not equally available everywhere.

You will, if you are traveling to a foreign country, want to check with the customs people also to see that you will be permitted to take your nonprescription medications along, what restrictions there may be if any, and also ask about bringing them back into our country.

If, as many people today do, you have a home away from home, it's an excellent idea to fit out each of your homes with those self-medication drug items that you'll need at that place. Now we are not talking only about a summer vacation place, for the chances are that you will stay at such a place for a sufficiently long time to warrant your moving your drug items with you. What we had in mind was a mobile home, a boat or camper or van. If you spend weekends in this secondary home, you might find it convenient to fit it out with your drug needs rather than having to *schlep* additionals each time.

The fact of the matter is that a vacation home will require certain medications that you do not use at your regular home, and vice-versa.

The greatest problem is that certain nonprescription medications you want will require refrigeration to prevent spoilage once the container is opened. You can't for example, put capsules into a case, toss them into the trunk of your car on a hot, sunny day, then expect to find capsules in the vial when you arrive at your destination.

The way we solve this problem is borrowed from the picnickers. Obtain a styrofoam picnic hamper with a tight-fitting lid. Put the drug supplies into this and then add a few of the commonly available frozen plastic ice packs. These plastic containers are filled with a glycerin-type chemical that is non-toxic. You put them into a freezer overnight, and the chemical freezes inside. While it takes longer to freeze than water does, the chemical also takes longer to thaw, is usually a good 12° colder than ordinary ice, and will turn that styrofoam hamper into a suitable refrigerator for at least twelve hours.

When you are ready to return home, simply refreeze the packets and they'll keep your medications (and even some fruits or containers of milk) nice and cold until you get home again.

It's far from pleasant to plan a fun-filled vacation and then to have to prepare for that unwanted medical problem as well. But things will indeed happen, especially while you're away from home, and the old adage that "an ounce of prevention is worth a pound of cure" isn't going to be much in the way of help. Part of vacation time celebrating is bound to be overeating, overexposure to the sun, and indulgence in everything you might avoid when you're at home. Taking the time to anticipate and prepare for the needs you may encounter while away can keep from spoiling the vacation you've been dreaming about.

Talking about vacations, it's a good idea to check with your physician and your pharmacist in the event that any recurring medical problems exist. Both the pharmacist and physician will be able to advise you of any special requirements that should be fulfilled before you leave.

Chapter Twenty

That Other Family Member

Most of us these days have pets, and our pets are as subject to medical problems as we are. Happily, when a pet animal becomes ill our usual practice is to rush it to a veterinarian for treatment. This is far better than the care we often offer ourselves.

When a pet has worked its way into your heart, you are prone to anthropomorphize, meaning that you imbue it with human qualities. How many times have you heard dog lovers talking to and about their dogs, saying "He says thank you." Actually, as cold and as hard as it may be to face, your pet is *not* human, it's an animal. It cannot communicate with you directly, but instead, learns that there are certain ways that you will understand its needs. When you've shared a home with a pet for any time at all, you will learn when it wants to go out. It has learned that sitting near the front door and whining will get you to open the door. After a time, you will come to recognize different signs and facial expressions. Your pet will soon have you "speaking its language."

It is our purpose here to discuss some of the problems to which pets are subject and show you how to cope with them.

When medication must be administered to a pet, there are several ways to do his. Liquids or powders can be mixed with some special food that the dog likes particularly. Where a medication must be given on a régular basis, it's a good idea to mix the medicine with some chopped meat and form this into small meatballs. These can then be frozen and allowed to thaw one at a time, as required for administration to the pet.

Pills, on the other hand, are another problem. Dogs are not all that stupid, and when you give a pill that's been concealed in a meatball, you will usually find that the dog will eat the meat and then spit out the pill.

The best way to feed a pill is to have the dog sit in front of you. Make it open its mouth by applying pressure with the fingers on the side of the jaw. When the jaws open, throw the pill in to the back of the throat, then with both hands hold the muzzle closed and pointing up. In a short time, you'll see the dog's tongue emerge from the front of the mouth, indicating that the pill has been swallowed. It works, and it works every time. After the pill has been swallowed, offer a small treat and a lot of praise. If you don't do this, getting the dog to hold still for the next pill feeding is going to be a problem.

Short of visiting a veterinarian, what can you do medically for your pet? Quite a bit, as it happens. We consulted for this information with Susan Wofsey, of Happicairn Kennels in Bethlehem, Connecticut.

Keep liquid or baby aspirin on hand, she advises, but only use this on the recommendation of your vet. Overdosage of aspirin can cause internal bleeding. Your vet will direct you when it has to be used and will tell you how much to use.

Remember that your dog is a lot closer to the ground than you are, and dust and sand can blow into the eyes. And some animals, especially French Poodles, are subject to eye irritation. Keep on hand a tube of eye ointment, but get the type with no Cortisone. This will ease eye irritation and can be used liberally. It's also a good idea to protect the animal's eye with this when shampooing it. By applying the eye ointment first, the irritating soap or detergent will not enter the eye and cause problems. Eyewash of the type that you would put in your own eyes can also be used.

A dog's nails have to be cut regularly, or the dog will be uncomfortable and will actually walk on its heels. The nerve in the nail, that black line that you see, will grow longer as the nail does. If you keep a dog's nails well trimmed, the nerve will recede so that you can cut them shorter each time, giving your dog added comfort. Use a standard dog nail clipper, cutting almost up to but not past the nerve.

You probably won't find it in a drugstore, but any pet shop will sell you a powder called Quik-Stop. It's technical name is Monsel's Solution, and it's used to stop bleeding immediately. This is needed when you are cutting a dog's nails and you cut too deeply. If you should do this, the Quick-Stop will stanch the bleeding.

Should your animal eat something it should not have ingested, and you require an emetic, use an ounce of hydrogen peroxide mixed with an ounce of water, but do this only on a vet's advice.

Should the animal have diarrhea or require an antacid, keep a supply of Kaobiotic Bolus medication on hand. You'll administer one tablet per nine pounds of body weight divided into two or three doses per day until the problem is corrected.

Occasionally your pet might step on something and cut its tender foot pad. This should be cleansed by a thorough soaking with hydrogen peroxide, and then a 2 percent solution of iodine should be applied. Naturally you'll want both of these products on hand for just such emergencies.

Keep a supply of Phisoderm liquid soap on hand, too. This is an antiseptic soap and is ideal for cleaning wounds or for washing tender or abraded skin.

Solarcain or some other antiseptic, analgesic spray should be available for minor cuts. This provides immediate pain relief, and as it is antiseptic, will counteract harmful bacteria.

Dogs are also subject to insect bites and stings. When it does happen, remember that as your pet is usually smaller than you are, the pain is more intense and the injected poisons even more harmful. Keep a small jar of Adolph's Meat Tenderizer on hand for such bites. Make a paste of the tenderizer and water and apply this liberally over the affected area. The pain will diminish almost at once, and you can almost see the swelling go down.

Should a minor burn occur, apply some Bacitracin ointment, available at any pharmacy.

If your dog spends any time in the outdoors, it's bound to be bitten by ticks and fleas. If you see it scratching or biting at its own skin, you can bet that this is the problem. Examine the animal carefully, pulling coat aside to see if you see any traces of these pests. If you should find one, spray a flea and tick killer directly on the insect, and then slowly and carefully pull the dead insect away. Many people simply yank the tick off, leaving the head under the dog's skin. This can result in infection later on. A little care and patience will go a long way toward keeping your pet comfortable.

If you travel with your pet, you may find that the animal is affected by motion sickness. It really does happen, and animals react just the way that kids do. They throw up and look very, very unhappy about the whole thing. Aside from this, most animals love to travel and consider it a real treat. If they see you heading for the family car, chances are that they will be in the car before you are.

Treating motion sickness requires a visit to your local pet shop, where you buy a package of Tranqua-Pet. Simply follow the package instructions and your dog will have no problems at all. Should you suspect that your pet is subject to motion sickness, to avoid the problem, administer this before embarking on a long trip as a preventive.

A word of caution is required here. Do not allow the dog to ride with its head out the window. Dogs really seem to love this, and on the surface it appears harmless enough. However, this is extremely bad for the dog's eyes and should not be permitted.

Do not leave your dog in a locked car with the windows up while you stop in for lunch at a restaurant. The rate of temperature elevation in a closed car on a sunny day is unbelievable, and you might well return to find a dead dog in the car. Rather, find a nice, shady spot, open the windows sufficiently so that air can circulate, but not so much that it can jump out and go looking for you. Remove its leash so that it cannot catch on something inside the car and strangle the animal.

If your animal is allowed to run free and there are rural areas around your home, you just might find it coming home one day smelling a bit ripe after an encounter with one of those little black pussycats with the white stripe down its back! Dogs are extremely curious, and seeing a skunk for the first time, your pet might offer some friendly overtures and come out on the short (and smelly) end of the stick. Skunks are not as gregarious as dogs are. Squirt! And it's all over. Now your pet comes running home, asking what you can do for it. Your first reaction might be to take your pet into the backyard and hose it down. Unfortunately, while this might cool it off, you still won't be able to get close to it. Skunk smell is insidious and long lasting.

What you have to do, believe it or not, is use tomato juice. Always keep a couple of gallons around for just such an emergency. It also works as well on humans who run into skunks.

Begin by applying the tomato juice undiluted all over the dog. Rub it in extremely well, covering the entire body. Allow this to sit and do its work for awhile, and then flush it all off. Now shampoo the dog with a 50-50 mixture of shampoo and tomato juice, wash that off, then shampoo again with straight shampoo.

Allow the dog to dry after washing the shampoo off, and you'll have your old sweet-smelling pet back once again, albeit a bit less anxious for another trek through the woods!

Pets chew furniture, especially when they're teething! Give them a suitable substitute for your furniture, such as a chewy bone, and that will stop. Cats like to claw furniture to pull and sharpen their claws. A kitty pole, covered with carpet can take the place of your furniture.

There are other things you could do. You could have the cat de-clawed. But have you ever seen how a de-clawed cat slinks along the baseboard near the wall? You've taken away its only defense and left it helpless. It's cruel and inhuman and not recommended.

Cats, too, have special problems and need periodic checking by a vet. Happily, when a cat is sick, it can let you know it. It will mope and keep pretty much to itself. If you see any such symptoms, or even more agonizing symptoms of any sort, get the poor cat to a vet, quick. If the cat seems to be preening itself too much, it might be dry skin, and a bit of fish oil in the food may help. An egg every other day will also keep the coat healthy. You can brush your cat too, and this grooming can be made a part of the affection you show the cat.

Remember that all animals have their own way to show gratitude and affection. To a cat, nothing is more valuable than a hunting trophy, so if your pet brings you a bird that it killed, it's showing gratitude. It won't understand your flying into a rage over it. Be a good sport, say "nice kitty" and then get rid of the bird as soon as its back is turned.

Cats also suffer from periodic hairballs, and a vet can diagnose and correct this. Have the animal checked for worms also.

Get the right shots when they are needed.

When something goes wrong with your pet, always begin with a call to your vet for his advice. Should he feel you should come in, he will tell you so. If the problem is a relatively minor one, he may suggest that you treat the animal at home. To do so, you're going to have certain medications on hand.

We hope this chapter will help.

Having a family pet is the end of loneliness, the beginning of love. Take care of your pet. You'll never regret it.

Introduction To Charts

In these charts you'll learn what and what not to take at the same time. Some of the words however require a bit of explanation.

A *contraindication* is a warning against taking the wrong medication for your problem. For example, if you have a splinter in your finger, you would not put a splint on it. By the same token, if you're a diabetic, any medication containing sugar might be contraindicated. Your family physician is best qualified to advise you on such matters.

Another important term is *interaction*. Some of the nonprescription drug items can interact with prescription drugs or other nonprescription drugs and either cancel out the hoped-for effects or possibly cause a great deal of harm.

The charts list the commonly available nonprescription drugs and also lists the ingredients that can be found in other drug products, both prescription and nonprescription.

If you are ill enough to need a prescription drug, you should tell your physician what nonprescription drugs you are presently taking so that he can advise you, if there is a possibility of a harmful interaction, to stop taking the nonprescription drug. Or ask your physician if it is all right to take a particular nonprescription drug you think might help. However, if for some reason you have not been able to ask your physician these questions, ask the pharmacist what the prescription drug contains, then check the list before buying a nonprescription drug to see if any interaction is possible. If so, don't buy the nonprescription drug.

If you're taking a nonprescription drug and want to take another, check the label carefully to see if any interaction may occur. If so, do not mix these items.

Interactions

PAIN KILLERS

If you take one of these	Avoid other products that contain
Alka-Seltzer	aspirin
Anacin	aspirin
Aspirin	aspirin
BC	aspirin
Bufferin	aspirin
Cope	aspirin, antihistamine
Doan's Pills	aspirin
Empirin Compound	aspirin
Excedrin	aspirin
Fizrin	aspirin
Midol	aspirin
Pamprin	antihistamines
Stanback	aspirin
Vanquish	aspirin

COUGH, COLD, ASTHMA

(inhaler products)

Asthmanefrin	sympathomimetic amines
Breatheasy	sympathomimetic amines
Bronkaid Mist	sympathomimetic amines
Primatene Mist	sympathomimetic amines

(liquids)

Coldene	antihistamines, aspirin, sympathomimetic amines
Robitussin -AC	antihistamines
Romilar CF	antihistamines, sympathomimetic amines
Super Anahist Cough Syrup	antihistamines
Terpin Hydrate, (also with Codeine, with Dextromethorphan)	alcohol

(nasal sprays or nose drops)

Contac	antihistamines, sympathomimetic amines
Neo-Synephrine	sympathomimetic amines
Privine	antihistamines
Sinex	antihistamines, sympathomimetic amines

If you take one of these	Avoid products that contain
St. Josephs Drops for Children	sympathomimetic amines
Super Anahist	antihistamines, sympathomimetic amines
(tablets and capsules) 4-Way Cold Tablets	aspirin, sympathomimetic amines
Allerest	antihistamines, sympathomimetic amines
Bromo-Quinine	sympathomimetic amines
Bronkaid	antihistamines, sympathomimetic amines
Cheracol Cold Capsules	antihistamines, aspirin sympathomimetic amines
Contac	antihistamines, sympathomimetic amines, belladonna alkaloids
Coricidin	antihistamines, aspirin,
Coricidin-D	antihistamines, aspirin, sympathomimetic amines
Coryban-D	antihistamines, sympathomimetic amines
Dristan	antihistamines, aspirin, sympathomimetic amines

SLEEP AIDS

Dormin	antihistamines
Nytol	antihistamines
Sleep-Eze	antihistamines, belladonna alkaloids
Sominex	antihistamines, belladonna alkaloids

ANTI-MOTION SICKNESS

Dramamine	antihistamines
Marezine	antihistamines
Mothersill's Remedy	belladonna alkaloids

Index

Absorption 147
Accessories 54-59
Acetaminophen 27, 69
Acne 97-99
Acute illness..................9
Additive reaction of drugs.......51
Adsorption 147
Aging, signs in medications 17
Aid, hearing 116-117
Alcohol.....................111
Alcohol, and anticoagulants 50
Alcohol, and drugs 39
Alcohol, contraindications against 41
Allergy 140-141
Allergies, drug................41
Aluminum 150
American Red Cross 83
Analgesics ..60-68, 70-71, 108, 133
Antacids 142-144, 149-157, 166-167
Antibiotics 64
Anticholinergics 125-127
Anticoagulants 50
Antidiarrheals 163-164
Antidotes for poisons...........57
Antiemetics 164, 165
Antihistamines ...125, 128-129, 131
Antipyretics 63
Antitussives 125
Aspirin .29, 60, 67-68, 69, 120, 181
Asthma 127, 128, 136
Athlete's foot 102-103
Axillary temperature.........62-63
Bandages 80, 86
Batteries, hearing aid 117-118
Bioavailability 16
Bidet........................56
Bites, dog....................83
Bleeding, treatment 84
Breathing 119, 136-139
Bruises, treatment...........85-88
Bronchodilators 125, 128

Buffering agent, purpose 20
Bulk-forming
  laxatives 161-162, 163
Burns 81-82, 89-95, 183
Calculus 110-111
Callouses 102
Capsules 18
Castor oil 145, 161
Cats, care of 184-185
Charcoal 133, 147-148
Chemical name of a drug 52
Children, administering
  medications to 32, 125
Children, and poisoning 23
Chloroform...................126
Chronic illness 9
Cleansing of wounds 85
Cold, common 122, 140-141
Combinations of drugs 39
Congeners...................148
Constipation 144-145
Contact lenses 115
Contraindications.....7, 40-41, 186
Controlled dosage medications 18-19
Cotton, absorbent..............22
Cough, types of 121
Cramp, muscle................171
Cumulative effect of dosages 30
Cumulative impact of drugs 51
Cuts 85-87, 182
Dandruff....................105
Dating medications 11
Decongestants
  ... 118, 125, 126, 127, 130, 131
Dehydrocholic acid 162
Dating medications 23
Dental care 109, 111
Dental floss 109
Dentures 109-110
Depressors, tongue 57
Deterioration of drugs 17-18

189

Diabetes 128
Diarrhea 145-146, 182
Digestion 142-169
"Discount drugs" 21
Disposing of medicines . . .13-14, 18
Dog bites .83
Dosage, completion of 33
Dosage control 43-44
Douche 56
Drug abuse 39
Drug interactions 48-53, 155
Dryness, skin 104
E, Vitamin 72, 73, 87
Ear .115-118
Eczema .102
Emergencies, first aid 78-83
Emetic 164, 165
Emetic, for animals 182
Endogenous pyrogens 63
Enema 55, 144, 157
Epidermis 96
Epinephrine 128
Exogenous pyrogens 63
Expectorants 125, 126, 127, 131
Eye 81, 113-115, 133-134
Eye cup 81, 114
Eyedrops 81, 113, 134
FDA .37-38
Federal Trade Commission 35
Fever 62-63, 120
Fever sores 103
First aid 78-83, 176
First-degree burns 89
Flatulence 147-148, 157
Flavored medications 32
Fleas, and animals 183
Food and Drug
    Administration . . .37-38, 122, 123
Food, Drug, and
    Cosmetic Act 123, 155
Foreign travel 175
Gallstones 142
Gargles .120
Gas .142-144

Gastric distress 45
Gastritis 142
Generic drug name 28, 53
Gingivitis 111
Glaucoma 114, 127
Glottis 138
Hair, ingrown 105
Hair, removal from nose 118
Hair, removal from ear 116
Hangover 148
Hay fever 128
Headache 64-67
Heath, Education, and Wel-
    fare, U.S. Department of . .34, 38
Hearing 115-116, 116-118
Heartburn 142-144
Heart disease 128
Heating pad 56
Hecht, Annabel 122
Hemorrhoids 103-104, 135
Hernia, hiatus 142
High blood pressure 128
Hoarseness 119
Hot-water bottle 55
Hydrophobia 83
Hyperacidity 142-144
Hyperosmotic laxatives 161, 162, 163
Hypertensive headache 65
Hypotention 50
Hypothalamus 63
Ice bag 55, 83
Impact injury 83, 88
Indigestion 142-144
Infarction, cardiac 142
Infarction, pulmonary 142
Inflammation 64
Ingrown toenail 106
Inhalers .136
Insect bites, and animals 182
Insert, package 34
Interactions, drug 48-53, 154, 187-188
Iodine, tincture of 79
Ipecac syrup 164
Irregularity 160

Itching, rectal 133
Itching, vaginal 132
Karate-ka 171
Kidneys 138
Labels, drug .22-23, 35, 40, 45, 123
Lactose 151
Laws regulating non-
    prescription drugs 35
Laxatives .144-145, 157-165, 168-169
Lenses, contact 115
Ligaments 170-171
Lips, chapped 106
Lobeline sulphate 138
Lozenges, throat 119
Lubricant laxatives 161, 163
Lungs 136-137
Magnesium 151
Mask, respirator 137
Medicine cabinet 8
Membranes, mucous 130-134
Membranes, swollen nasal 136
Mercurochrome 79
Merthiolate, tincture of 79
Metabolism of drugs 50
Migraine 65
Mineral oil 145, 162
Minimum Adult
    Daily Requirements 72
Minor burns 89
Motion sickness 146, 183
Mouth 107-112, 131-132
Mouthwash 109, 110, 112
Mucosal erosion of mouth ... 67-68
Mucous membranes 130-134
Multivitamins 72
Muscles 170-174
Muscle tonus 146
N.F. 37
Names, types for drugs ... 28, 52-53
National Formulary 37
"Natural" laxative 159
Nausea 146
Nicotine 138
Nose 88, 118-119

Nose drops 131
OTC Drug Review 156, 158
OTC drugs 11, 34
Odor, foot 103
Off-brand medications 28
Oiliness, skin 104-105
Ointments, muscle 172-173
Opiates 164
Oral temperature 62
Overdosing 11, 68
Over-the-counter drugs 11, 34
Oxygen equipment 57
Package inserts 8
Pain 60-61
Pain, minor 61-62
Pancreatitis 142
Patent remedies 11
Peroxide, hydrogen 79, 80
Pets..................... 180-185
Pharmacist 35, 43
Phenobarbital 129
Pills, and animals 181
Pilonidal cyst 105
Poison antidotes 57
Poison Prevention Packaging Act .37
Poisoning, aspirin 68
Polycarbophil 164
Pores 96
Potassium 151
Prescription drugs 36, 178
Private label drugs 29
Proprietary Association 26
Proprietary name 53
Prostate gland, enlargement of .. 128
Psoriasis 100-101, 105
Psychogenic headache 66
Punctures.................. 84-85
Pure Food and Drug laws 28
Pyrogens 63
Quality-control sampling 22
Quantities of
    medications to purchase 15
Radio-frequency burns 92
Razor cuts 87

191

Reactions 36, 41, 45-47
Rectal temperature 62
Rectum 133
Red Cross, American 83
Redness of the eye 113
Refrigeration of drugs 10, 179
Relining of dentures 109
Respirator mask 137
Restocking of medicines 20-27
Rheumatic conditions 64
Safety packaging 19, 37
Saline laxatives 161, 162, 163
Salivary glands 131
Scalds 81-82, 89-95
Scales, bathroom 58-59
Scaling of teeth 110-111
Scissors, bandage 56-57
Scrapes 84, 87
Scratches 84
Seasickness 146
Seborrhea 105
Second-degree burns 82, 89
Self-medication 10-11
Shingles 102
Side effects 36, 46-48
Skin 96-106
Skunks, removing odor of 184
Slivers, removal 80-81
Smoking 138-139
Snakebites 82
Snoring 137-138
Sodium 151, 160-161
Solubility 16
Sore throat 119-121
Sores, fever 103
Spasm, muscle 171
Spansules 44, 122
Sphygmomanometer 57
Splinters, removal 80-81
Splints 82
Spoons, measuring 31
Stethoscope 57
Stimulant laxatives 161, 162, 163
Stings, insect 82-83
Stomach 24, 142-169

Stool softener laxatives 161, 163
Stopples, ear 116
Stuffers 7
Stuffiness of nose 118-119
Styptic 87
Sunburn 82, 89, 90-92, 95
Suppositories 144, 163
Suppressants, cough 127
Swabs, cotton 57, 81
Tablets, signs of deterioration 18
Tartar 110-111
Teeth 107-111
Temperature, body 62-63
Tendons 170-171
Tetanus 79, 83, 85, 87
Tetracycline 150
Thermometers 54-55
Third-degree burns 82, 89
Throat 119-121
Thyroid disease 128
Ticks, and animals 183
Timed-release
   cold formulations 124-125
Tincture 9
Toenail, clipping of dog's . . . 181-182
Toenail, ingrown 106
Tongue 132
Tongue depressors 57
Toxic vascular headache 66
Trachea 136-137
Trauma 83
Tweezers 80-81
U.S.P. 37
United States Pharmacopeia 37
Vaginal itching 132
Vaporizers 56, 119, 131, 139
Vapors, noxious 137
Vitamin poisoning 72
Vitamins 72-77, 87, 111, 129
Warnings, antacid 153
Warts 101-102
Water in ear 116
Wax, ear 81, 115
Worms 133
Wounds 79-81, 84-88